Mastering Menopause

Mastering Menopause

Women's Voices on Taking
Charge of the Change

Deborah M. Merrill

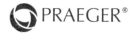 PRAEGER®

An Imprint of ABC-CLIO, LLC
Santa Barbara, California • Denver, Colorado

Library of Congress Cataloging-in-Publication Data

Names: Merrill, Deborah M., 1962- author.
Title: Mastering menopause : women's voices on taking charge of the change
  / Deborah M. Merrill.
Description: Santa Barbara, California : Praeger, an imprint of ABC-CLIO, LLC, [2020] |
  Includes bibliographical references and index.
Identifiers: LCCN 2019037263 (print) | LCCN 2019037264 (ebook) | ISBN
  9781440874710 (hardcover) | ISBN 9781440874727 (ebook)
Subjects: LCSH: Menopause—Psychological aspects. | Middle-aged
  women—Attitudes. | Life change events.
Classification: LCC RG186 .M488 2020 (print) | LCC RG186 (ebook) | DDC
  618.1/75—dc23
LC record available at https://lccn.loc.gov/2019037263
LC ebook record available at https://lccn.loc.gov/2019037264

ISBN: 978-1-4408-7471-0 (print)
      978-1-4408-7472-7 (ebook)

24 23 22 21 20   1 2 3 4 5

This book is also available as an eBook.

Praeger
An Imprint of ABC-CLIO, LLC

ABC-CLIO, LLC
147 Castilian Drive
Santa Barbara, California 93117
www.abc-clio.com

This book is printed on acid-free paper ∞

Manufactured in the United States of America

This book is for the women who so generously
shared their lives with me,
Wendy O'Leary and the members of my
Monday-morning sangha,
and for Ken, always.

Not all of us are called to be hermits, but all of us need enough silence and solitude in our lives to enable the deeper voice of our own self to be heard.

—Thomas Merton

It is like you come out on the other side of menopause and life is so, so much better.

—Anonymous

Contents

Acknowledgments

This book would not have been possible without the assistance of the fifty women who generously shared their time and their lives with me. They graciously revealed their innermost thoughts and feelings at one of the most difficult times of their lives. I will always be grateful for the opportunity to hear their stories and share their journeys. Their identities have been changed in this book to preserve their privacy. All the women have been given pseudonyms and are presented as a composite of several women.

This book would also not have been possible without the generous funding of Clark University. I am indebted to the Research Board and Office of Research and Graduate Studies for awarding me a Faculty Development Grant to provide the respondents with a stipend for their time. Such a stipend legitimizes studies like mine and makes it more likely that respondents will participate. I am grateful to my colleagues at Clark for their continued confidence in my work.

I would also like to thank the members of the sociology department at Clark for their support, collegiality, and friendship. Most of us have worked together for more than twenty-five years, and we have shared all the ups and downs of life. I am particularly grateful to Shelly Tenenbaum, who chaired the department so that I could chair the faculty for three years *and* take a semester sabbatical to write a rough draft of the book. Shelly has been a stalwart supporter and role model over the years, and I admire and appreciate her greatly. I chose my position at Clark twenty-seven years ago because of my colleagues, and I have never regretted the decision.

Many thanks to my friend and pastor, Reverend Aaron Payson, who supports and encourages me and others to live an undivided life. Aaron and all my friends at the Unitarian Universalist Church of Worcester have brought great meaning to my life and given me the tools to live authentically. A comedy of errors led me to the UUCW, but it was the best mistake of my life.

Finally, my thanks to my students, who make it a joy to go to work every day. It is a privilege to know you and to work with you, and I am grateful to be your professor. Thank you for the integrity and authenticity you bring to the classroom and, most importantly, for being you.

I would also like to thank my editor, Debbie Carvalko, for believing in my work once again.

ONE

Introduction

I made an appointment to see a therapist because I had been feeling depressed. One of the first questions that she asked me was how old I was. I said 52. She said, "You are probably perimenopausal. Many women experience depression as they go through menopause because of unresolved issues that come to light around hormonal changes." Menopause? Me? Menopause? It had never occurred to me. I was old enough . . . in theory . . . but it just never entered my mind that I could be going through menopause.

—Cynthia, fifty-six years of age

Menopause strikes many women from out of the blue, like Cynthia above. Their menstrual cycle becomes erratic, or they suddenly stop menstruating altogether. They do not automatically think of perimenopause or menopause, though. They may even experience some of the symptoms, such as erratic periods or irritability, without attributing it to "the change." Those women who experience regular hot flashes are more likely to know what is happening to their bodies as this symptom is almost always associated with menopause. How women experience menopause, how they treat the symptoms, and what meaning they give to menopause are the subjects of this book. Each of these is expected to vary considerably across women according to class, race, educational level, and culture. Based on extensive interviews with women who are either perimenopausal or postmenopausal, this book will provide a comprehensive picture of women's menopausal experiences today.

Unlike other books on menopause, this book is rich in the details of women's lived experiences. Through the extensive use of quotations throughout the book, it is written in the women's own words. The book also includes information on the most up-to-date advice on treating symptoms, according to both researchers and the women going through menopause. The topic of menopause is important because it affects every aspect of women's midlife period: their health, sex lives, relationships with family, and how they feel about themselves. The menopausal years are a time when many women address the unresolved issues of earlier life that they have not had time to examine. It is a juncture when they reprioritize their lives and their choices of how to spend their time. Women learn how to cope with potentially debilitating symptoms and decide how they wish to live the second half of their adult years.

BACKGROUND ON MENOPAUSE

Menopause, sometimes called "the change," refers to the time in a woman's life when menstrual periods stop permanently and the woman is no longer able to bear children. The average age at which menopause occurs is forty-nine to fifty-two years of age. The permanent cessation to menstruation is said to have occurred when a woman has not had any vaginal bleeding for one full year. There may be several occurrences of months without menstruation followed by a period before a woman reaches a final full year without a period. This type of irregularity is common. However, a full twelve-month cessation from the last menstrual cycle is required to be defined as menopausal.[1,2] (Please see Appendix A: Glossary of Menopause-Related Terminology.)

Menopausal symptoms tend to be worse early in menopause. The beginning of menopause, referred to as perimenopause or "around" menopause, usually occurs anywhere between two and eight years, but can occur ten to twelve years, prior to menopause. Menopausal symptoms tend to decrease and then cease within one year or so after a woman's last period. Overall, the duration of menopause (from the start of perimenopause to the end of one full year without a period) usually lasts five to ten years but may take as many as thirteen to fifteen years. A few women will continue to have at least some menopausal symptoms such as hot flashes for as many as twenty years postmenopause.[3]

Menopause occurs due to a decrease in hormone production by the ovaries. Prior to menopause, periods will be irregular, both in timing and length. Although the severity of symptoms varies, most women experience "hot flashes" that last anywhere between thirty seconds and ten minutes, vaginal dryness, mood swings, and trouble sleeping. Some women have not had any symptoms when they realize they have not experienced a period for over one year. Menopause typically occurs naturally, that is, without any intervention. However, it may also occur as the result of the removal of both ovaries (referred to as a full hysterectomy) or usage of some types of chemotherapy. As a result, menopause may occur in some women in their thirties.[4,5,6]

Prior to menopause, a woman's ovaries decrease production of the hormone progesterone, followed by the hormone estrogen. The imbalance of the two hormones makes the symptoms of perimenopause more severe than later in the menopausal trajectory. Symptoms of menopause can most effectively be addressed by a combined estrogen/progesterone treatment referred to as estrogen replacement therapy (ERT) or hormone replacement therapy (HRT). However, because of the increased risk of breast cancer as a result of HRT, physicians prefer to prescribe it only when there are extreme or life-altering symptoms, and then only in very low doses for a short period. This does not always coincide with a woman's perception of her need for HRT. That is, some women may request HRT even when their physicians do not see it as warranted. Women who wish to verify that they are going through menopause may have a urine or blood test to check for the presence of the follicle-stimulating hormone (FSH), which increases during menopause, as well as estrogen (or estradiol), which decreases during menopause. The number of hormones begins to change prior to menopause, when there are often other symptoms present as well. This time period, referred to as perimenopause, may be as long as a six-year phase of irregular periods, hot flashes, sleep disturbance, night sweats, and mood swings. Some women continue to experience symptoms fifteen to twenty years after menopause. Women who have ceased menstruating for one or more years are referred to as postmenopausal, even if they continue to experience side effects.[7,8,9,10]

Symptoms and Treatments

The most common side effects of menopause include hot flashes[11] (occurring in 41 percent to 75 percent of women); insomnia (33 percent of women); vaginal atrophy due to loss of lubrication, which makes intercourse painful[12] (75 percent of women); fatigue and lack of energy

(50 percent of women); irritability (41 percent); and night sweats[13] (33 percent).[14,15,16,17] Symptoms tend to be more severe during perimenopause and then subside as women get closer to menopause. Until 2002, estrogen/progesterone supplements (also referred to as hormone replacement therapy, or HRT) were a common treatment prescribed by physicians for severe hot flashes, insomnia, night sweats, and painful intercourse caused by vaginal atrophy and dryness. HRT was the most effective treatment for what were often debilitating symptoms.

However, physicians and researchers were concerned about the potential side effects of this treatment throughout its usage. In 1991 the National Institutes of Health and National Institute of Heart, Lung, and Blood started the Women's Health Initiative, a multimillion-dollar longitudinal study lasting over twenty years, to look at the major health issues in postmenopausal women. It was the largest study of women's health, with a sample size of 161,808 women. Several clinical trials were part of the overall study, including one that examined the impact of hormone replacement therapy (estrogen alone and combined estrogen and progestin [Prempro™]) on 68,132 postmenopausal women aged fifty to seventy-nine years. In addition, there was an observational study of 93,000 women, which followed their medical histories and health habits.

The trial continued for over a decade before the disclosure of critical findings. The study found that trial participants using the combined estrogen and progesterone supplement showed increased risk of heart disease, breast cancer, stroke, and blood clots among previously healthy women. These results were published in 2002 in the *Journal of the American Medical Association* and were widely disseminated from there. The authors cited a 26 percent increase in breast cancer risk for women, particularly for those who had been taking estrogen/progestin for a longer period of time. Recipients of the combined hormone also had higher rates of heart disease, stroke, and blood clots.

Following the 2002 study, many women discontinued use of estrogen/progestin resulting in decreases in breast cancer by as early as 2003.[18] Other studies have found, however, that use of estrogen alone does not increase risk of breast cancer for women with a prior hysterectomy.[19] Most physicians now caution women to use estrogen/progesterone in the smallest doses possible over a short period of time to address only extreme cases of hot flashes, night sweats, insomnia, and other symptoms.[20,21]

However, some women do continue to use HRT today to lessen menopausal symptoms. Even more women may request HRT without receiving it. One of the goals of this study is to examine under what conditions women may request and use HRT despite knowing the potential side effects. Do they make this request only when symptoms are debilitating and they have no other choice, or do they seek relief under less severe conditions as well? In addition, is the choice to request HRT related to a medical meaning attached to menopause, or do they seek hormone supplements even with nonmedical constructions of menopause?

There are other, longer-term side effects of menopause. Osteoporosis and heart disease risk both increase in women following menopause due to the decrease in estrogen levels.[22] This is particularly significant as heart disease is the leading cause of death among women fifty years of age and older in America. Heart disease accounts for 22.3 percent of deaths among women fifty years of age and over, followed by cancer deaths at 21.1 percent.[23]

Pharmacological Treatments

Other pharmacological treatments include the use of selective serotonin reuptake inhibitors (SSRIs) and serotonin-norepinephrine reuptake inhibitors (SNRIs). SSRIs and SNRIs increase levels of serotonin and norepinephrine, both neurotransmitters, in the brain and are typically used to treat depression and anxiety. Neurotransmitters affect communication in brain nerve cell circuitry. Both neurotransmitters have been found to reduce hot flashes and night sweats and improve the quality of sleep.[24,25] SSRIs increase the level of serotonin solely in the brain by blocking its reabsorption, but they have fewer side effects. SNRIs block the reabsorption of both neurotransmitters. SSRIs and SNRIs both require a doctor's prescription. More information on the use of SSRIs and SNRIs is included in Chapter 2.

Women can also take bioidentical hormones to treat symptoms of menopause. Bioidentical hormones are synthesized from natural products, typically plants, to produce the identical structure of the hormones produced by the human body. It is this identical structure that medically trained specialists believe make them particularly effective. They further believe that their "natural" or plant-based source make them safer, but it is not clear whether they are any safer than hormones produced in a lab. The hormones are produced in different formats (creams and lotions, injections, tablets, etc.) and concentrations.[26,27,28] Some bioidentical hormones are regulated by the Food and Drug Administration, whereas others produced in compounding pharmacies are not regulated. Most require a prescription. Although they have been found to reduce hot flashes and vaginal dryness, the potential consequences of prolonged usage are not known. This is due to the variety of formats, concentrations, and sources of creation. Some reported side effects include heart disease, breast cancer, stroke, and risk of blood clots.[29] How these bioidentical hormones work to relieve menopausal symptoms and the better-known products will be discussed in the next chapter.

Not all women are aware of the effectiveness of antidepressants in treating menopause or the availability of bioidentical hormones. This book will examine under what conditions women turn to these pharmacological interventions and whether or not their usage is related to a medical construction of menopause. It is assumed that women typically do not learn of these treatments until they see a physician. Some may be reluctant to use an antidepressant or to risk using a bioidentical hormone. The influence of the physician in making this decision will shed light on the continued role of medicine in the menopause experience.

Lifestyle Changes and Other Natural Remedies

Although not presented as a cure-all for the symptoms of menopause, there are known benefits from exercise, proper diet, and limiting alcohol and caffeine.[30,31] Exercise helps to control the weight gain that comes with reduced metabolism; reduces risk of high blood pressure, heart attacks, and strokes; improves sleep; and reduces depression, anxiety, and stress.[32,33] Limiting alcohol also helps to keep calories under control, and reducing caffeine intake helps to ensure adequate sleep. A proper diet, which includes low-fat proteins, soy, vegetables, whole grains, and limited fruit, all optimize the body's natural functioning.[34,35,36,37] Calcium and vitamin D are suggested to minimize risk of osteoporosis. Vitamin B complex and vitamin E are also encouraged. Vitamin B helps to transform food into energy; assists the cardiovascular, immune, and nervous systems; works with the brain to produce serotonin and norepinephrine to improve mood and decrease irritability; and produces melatonin to aid sleep. Vitamin E is taken for optimal cardiovascular health. This is particularly important for postmenopausal women as heart disease is the number-one cause of death in postmenopausal women. Combined, these lifestyle choices optimize older women's health in general, including those undergoing menopause.

One of the goals of this book is to examine the conditions under which women use these lifestyle changes to control the symptoms of menopause.

It is expected that future generations of women will be more likely to turn to diet, exercise, and lifestyle changes in response to menopause. However, these changes are unlikely to make a large impact when menopausal symptoms are severe. What tradeoffs women make when lifestyle change is not enough to combat symptoms is one among many of the questions asked in this book.

Another important alternative to estrogen replacement therapy for women is the consumption of phytoestrogens, which are found in plants but act like the estrogen in one's body. Nature is full of theses estrogen mimickers. In particular, they are found in soy, black cohosh, dong quai, ginseng, and red clover. Medical journals, however, state that the estrogen mimickers have not all been proven to be effective. What has been found to be effective in reducing hot flashes, night sweats, and vaginal dryness, however, is soy, but women must consume at least 160 mg per day in order for it to be effective. This is essentially three servings of soy per day. In a randomized, double-blind study of ninety-three women, effects were seen twelve weeks following consumption of soy at this level.[38]

Acupuncture can also play a role in relieving the symptoms of menopause. It has been shown to have a positive effect on the production and circulation of hormones in the body. This ensures that neurotransmitters, such as serotonin and norepinephrine, are in balance, which then creates a greater sense of well-being and calm.[39]

The use of phytoestrogens, acupuncture, and Eastern practices such as yoga may be effective, but they are not commonly or traditionally used to treat menopause. It is expected that current and future generations of women, particularly more educated young women, may be more likely to consider them. It is hypothesized that this is part of a general trend of treating menopause with psychospiritual treatments rather than pharmacological treatments such as hormone replacement. It is further hypothesized that younger women will use meditation and perhaps therapy in a quest to make the menopausal period one of personal growth and examination of unresolved issues that come up during menopause. This possibility will be discussed further below.

Menopause: A Time of Change

Menopause is often referred to as "the change" because of the transition women experience from being fertile to infertile. However, many women believe that they change during menopause in other ways as well. They view menopause as a "marker" and "passage" that results in positive change in their lives overall.[40] In previous research, women explained that the changes in their bodies force them to reexamine their lives. Women without children see menopause as an even more significant marker of important life transitions than those with children, as they do not have other markers, such as having their offspring graduate from school or marry. In a previous study, one woman said, "[It is a] turning point to live life the way you really want to live without compromising as much as before."[41] Similarly, another woman said that menopause created an opportunity to take a different career path. A third woman saw it as a new beginning. She said that she was excited about the way her life was going and that she got to do more of what she wanted to do. Overall, women talked about menopause helping them to recognize the importance of building good support systems and of reexamining friendships, other significant relationships, and how they spent their time. One woman said, "It encourages you to begin to concentrate and care for yourself. Most of the rest of life we are . . . care giving."[42] Others said that it increased their sense of personal power and was an opportunity to exercise new freedoms, such as spending time on things that they really enjoyed. More than half of the women saw it as a marker of getting older. Still, they saw this in a positive light. It gave them a new sense of wisdom and an opportunity for self-understanding that they did not have earlier.

Gail Sheehy, well-known author of the blockbuster *Passages*,[43] which examines the changes in men and women's lives over the life course, and its successor, *The Silent Passage Menopause*,[44] states that more changes take place during this passage called menopause than at any other point in an adult woman's life. She argues that women change in relation to themselves and others and use this time to consider a new sense or way of being. They may reprioritize how they spend their time and thus reconsider their careers, marriages, and relationships with others. They may even "reinvent" who they are. Sheehy sees this as a very positive time for women, referring to it as "busting out" and "living out the fantasy."

What is it about menopause that causes this psychological reflection? Many of the women felt "out of control" or vulnerable in ways they had not before menopause. One woman described how her body was taking a different shape in front of her eyes. She felt more uncertain in life, due in part to erratic periods and hot flashes. Women said that they had to learn to be more flexible because of unpredictable periods starting and that they found themselves "tearing up" or weeping without warning. Their vulnerability, caused by heavy periods and intense emotions, made them more open to change. For example, some women said that menopause caused them to rethink their decisions about childbearing. That is, some regretted never having children. Three of the women talked about "turning inward" as a result of menopause. One woman said that she felt more connected to her inside self, even though she thought her body was out of control. She said, "I really know who I [am] and what I [am] feeling."[45] Another woman said that feeling out of control caused her to pull away from others and want to be left alone. She had previously been very social, however. In contrast, other women became more spiritual out of a desire to be part of a bigger picture.

In addition, our brains change at perimenopause. A switch goes on at this time that signals alteration in the temporal lobe, which is the site of long-term memory and enhanced intuition. During perimenopause, there is a complex interaction between the hypothalamus, pituitary gland, ovaries, and the hormones GnRH (gonadotropin-releasing hormone), FSH (follicle-stimulating hormone), estrogen, and progesterone. The hypothalamus is responsible for motivational behaviors and is key for experiencing and expressing emotions. It regulates the production of these hormones and is regulated by them. Reproductive hormones are directly responsible for stimulating opioid centers in the brain that make nurturing pleasurable when women are in their child-rearing years. However, the decrease in these hormones during perimenopause allows other interests to surface in sharper focus and allows us to understand and express anger that was not there before during perimenopause and menopause. The rewiring of a woman's brain makes her thoughts clearer and her motivations easier to identify. Tending to emotions when one becomes aware of them is critical because of the connections between the brain, the heart and cardiovascular system, the immune system, and other organs and physiological systems. Not attending to emotional needs eventually leads to somatic diseases.[46]

In previous studies, women reexamined their relationships with spouses during menopause. Perhaps more importantly, they also reexamined those relationships because of their husband's role in their menopausal experience. For example, many of the women were disappointed if their husbands were not willing to find out more about menopause and discuss it with them. They wanted their husbands to understand what they were experiencing. One woman said that recognizing her husband's lack of interest in her experience played a significant role in her decision to leave him at that time. Other women believed that their husbands were critical of their mood swings and irritability. Only a few of the married women said that their husbands had been supportive and responsive. For example, one husband brought his wife books about menopause and encouraged her to discuss them with him. In contrast, all but one of the single women said that it would have been easier to negotiate menopause if they had a long-term intimate partner with whom they could share reactions and feelings.[47]

Physician Christiane Northrup points out that relationship crises and the need to confront unresolved conflict from the past are a common side effect of menopause. She explains, "These hormone-driven changes affect the brain, they give a woman a sharper eye for inequity and injustice, and a voice that insists on speaking up about them . . . they uncover hidden wisdom—and the courage to voice it."[48] Northrup points out that stresses and unresolved problems or long-sublimated desires that simmered beneath the surface during child-rearing years bubble up and boil over at perimenopause. Health problems manifest if women do not face the changes they need to make or resolve the conflict. This may include uncovering unconscious and self-destructive beliefs and patterns about oneself and one's relationships and addressing unhealed hurts. "Our hormones are giving us an opportunity to see, once and for all, what we need to change in order to live honestly, fully, joyfully, and healthfully in the second half of our lives."[49] Though it may be the hormonal fluctuations that initially bring the distress to the surface, how this affects us depends on whether we notice these new thoughts and our ability and willingness to make changes in our lives.

How does this unresolved conflict lead to poor health for women? Emotions that feel bad are trying to get our attention so that we can either change our behavior or our perception to alter those emotions. Unresolved emotions keep getting "stuck" and setting up the same biochemical response, which eventually causes an escalation in the stress response. Throughout much of perimenopause, estrogen is *high* before it drops in late perimenopause, causing serotonin to drop as well. When serotonin drops, the neurotransmitter norepinephrine spikes; the body perceives this as stress and produces cortisol. High levels of cortisol over long periods result in cardiovascular disease and a condition referred to as "chronic stress."[50]

This stress response, however, does not have to occur. According to Dr. Christiane Northrup, "health is enhanced by allowing all emotions to wash in and out like the tides of the sea. At midlife, sadness and regrets from our past take on a heightened role for a time . . . helping us

to clean up our emotional lives . . . and setting the stage for more fulfill-
ment and joy to come in."[51] The most significant way of contributing to
our own good health is through recognition of our thoughts and emotions. Menopause and changes in the midlife brain allow us to step back,
acknowledge the need for change, and separate from long-term destructive life patterns. This allows women to emerge from menopause with a
greater understanding of themselves and the need for any change in
their lives.

How, though, do women recognize these emotions and the need for
change? One of the prominent themes of this book is the importance of
utilizing meditation and mindfulness in recognizing difficult emotions
that are highlighted at menopause and working through those emotions to
resolve them. Menopause can bring great joy to a woman's life if she is
able to resolve earlier conflicts or reprioritize things to make her life run
more smoothly. With a greater understanding of her own needs and the
way to meet them, a woman may find that menopause can be a gateway to
a more joyful second half of life.

A Broad Range of Experiences

As one of the women in this book stated, "Menopause is hard." It can
come out of the blue. A woman may be well into perimenopause before
she even realizes that she is menopausal. Usually it is irritating or debilitating symptoms that lead her to a doctor and thus a diagnosis of perimenopause. In addition to the physical symptoms of hot flashes, insomnia,
fatigue, night sweats, and vaginal dryness, women may also experience
depression and mood swings. Many reflect on where they have been and
where they wish to go in their lives.

However, not all women experience physical symptoms. A few of the
women said that they discovered they were perimenopausal when they
woke up one morning and realized that it had been months since they had
a period. They went on to suffer no physical symptoms throughout menopause, but they did give greater thought to their priorities. Thus, there is a
wide range of experiences, with some women having no physical symptoms while others experience intense hot flashes as often as every twenty
minutes.

The onset of menopause also varies considerably. Women who underwent a hysterectomy or who took certain medications for cancer were
plunged into menopause during their thirties. In contrast, the average age

of entering "natural" menopause is forty-nine to fifty-two years of age. The women in this study had all gone through menopause by the age of fifty-five years old. However, some women experienced hot flashes and insomnia through their sixties. One woman was seventy-nine years of age and still experiencing hot flashes. It will be argued in this book that women's experience of menopause has much to do with the meaning that they attribute to it.

Finally, women varied in the meaning they attributed to menopause. While some focused on the implications of menopause for their femininity and sexual appeal, others saw it as a liberation from the constraints of birth control and having young children. Many were concerned with the implications for their appearance while others were thinking about what they could do now that they did not have to worry about starting their periods. For many it was a period of rebirth and a second chance to "get it [their lives] right." Others saw menopause as an extension of having periods and pregnancies, all of which are interconnected parts of being women.

OUTLINE OF THE BOOK

The purpose of this book is to look at how the social meaning of menopause has changed over time. Prior to the twentieth century, menopause was seen as a normal part of a woman's life. However, menopause became medicalized during the twentieth century. That is, it was seen as a physiological deficiency to be treated with pharmaceutical intervention. This was further reinforced when authors Wilson and Wilson[52] claimed that menopause defeminized women and that they needed to turn to HRT to regain their femininity. It will be argued in this book that menopause is once again seen as a normal part of the life course but that women now expect some sort of assistance in treating the physical symptoms as well as the psychological ones that come with menopause and changes in the brain. It will be argued that women today are seeking a spiritual/psychological solution and are turning to meditation and mindfulness to get them through their menopausal years. They are also looking to treat symptoms with a well-balanced diet supplemented with phytoestrogens, exercise, limited caffeine and alcohol, and other lifestyle changes.

This book will also look at the broad range of social meanings that women attribute to menopause and how its social construction affects their experience. We will look at how the social locations produced by different levels of education, race, and culture thus affect women's experiences through the meanings they hold for menopause. The history of black women's relationship with the medical community will play an important role in this discussion.

Throughout the book, I argue that menopause often holds negative meanings for women. For some, menopause is a loss of their femininity. For others, it is far worse than they expected it to be. Yet, menopause also holds the opportunity for significant personal growth and renewal when women take the opportunity to look deeply at the emotions that spring to the surface and make the changes that will bring greater joy to the second half of their lives. Seeing these emotions and working through them is much more likely with meditation and mindfulness and, in some instances, therapy. While the journey may be long, the payoff will be tremendous.

Chapter 2 will examine the portrayal of menopause in the media and the history of treating menopause, including a deeper discussion of treatment today. The portrayal of menopause in the media is likely to affect women's social construction of it, given the pervasiveness of the media in our lives. Understanding how menopause has been treated in the past and how it is treated today are also important in comprehending how women perceive menopause and how it is socially constructed. Women began experiencing menopause when they lived longer than their reproductive years. By 1901, women's average life expectancy reached 52.4 years of age, allowing most women to experience menopause.[53]

Chapter 3 provides a detailed discussion of women's experiences in their own words. This includes their use of physicians, their expectations of menopause, and the existence of support networks where the networks occur. It includes the type, severity, and length of symptoms and how women have treated them. This chapter also gives examples of surgically induced menopause and discusses how it may differ from "natural" menopause. It is important to validate the range of women's experiences in order to normalize their particular circumstances.

Chapter 4 will be the first of two chapters that look at the social meaning of menopause, both in the literature and what was found in this study. It will highlight the impact of education on women's menopausal experience and how education informs different social meanings. In particular, it will show how less-educated women experience menopause much more negatively because they see it as a loss of the things that matter most to them as women: their sex appeal and their ability to have children. It will also look at the benefits that better-educated women associate with menopause and the circumstances under which women use HRT.

Chapter 5 is the second chapter to examine the impact of the social meaning of menopause. In this chapter, I consider black and Latina women's experiences of menopause. The chapter will focus on the impact of black women's history on their perception of the medical community today and the implications for menopause. The impact of Latinx culture on menopause will also be discussed. This chapter will support the argument that race still matters in the United States in the twenty-first-century.

Chapter 6 looks at women's psychosocial needs at menopause and how mindfulness and meditation can be used both to manage symptoms better and to make beneficial life changes. The chapter includes a discussion of the need for mindfulness at menopause, in particular, and provides examples of the kinds of life changes the women in this study made.

Chapter 7 examines the impact of menopause overall on marriage, women's sex lives, and their relationships with extended family. Like all the other chapters, this too is written in the women's own words.

Chapter 8 goes into greater detail in explaining how meditation assists women in addressing difficult emotions, letting go of story lines and obsessive thinking, learning to live in the present moment and accept things as they are, and to recognize that our thoughts are not necessarily truth and how that can lead to reconciliation. Three case studies with varying degrees of meditation usage are discussed.

Chapter 9 summarizes the findings and discusses implications.

TWO

Popular Culture and a History of Treating Menopause

POPULAR CULTURE AND MENOPAUSE

Popular culture, like the medical community, has constructed menopause as a solely biological or physiological event and a negative period of loss. Betty Friedan, in her book *The Fountain of Age*, documents the scarcity of older women (sixty years of age and older) in the media in the late twentieth century.[1] She refers to this paucity of older persons in television, film, magazine, and society in general as the "denial of aging."[2] She argues that menopause should not be seen as a disease that needs to be cured but instead should be seen as another stage of life with opportunities for meaningful engagement in society. She maintains that there is a new "brouhaha" surrounding menopause that stresses its difficulties, something she sees as unfortunate. By saying this, though, she undermines what can be a debilitating and upending period of a woman's life. She stated that those women who experience any kind of "trauma" in menopause are allowing themselves to be defined strictly by their biological role. As will be seen in this book, the symptoms of menopause can be severe enough to warrant trauma for many women. It should be noted that Freidan's very popular book was published a decade before researchers detailed the significant impact of HRT on the risk of breast cancer (to be discussed later in the chapter). With no alternative as effective as HRT, she could not predict the bind that women would be in without a safe treatment for oppressive and debilitating hot flashes, night sweats, and insomnia, among other symptoms. The message of her book was that popular culture overinflates the difficulty of menopause while also denying the aging process in America.

In contrast was the message given by another well-known author, Gail Sheehy, author of the bestselling *Passages* and *The Silent Passage: Menopause*. In the latter book, she presents the range of menopause symptoms and the potential for a stressful, emotional time, with hot flashes that may send a woman fleeing to her physicians. While not all women will know each symptom, this book prepares women for the potential difficulties they may encounter.[3]

There are no popular films that focus on menopause. There have been sitcoms with episodes devoted to menopause, though. *All in the Family* was the first such sitcom. In the episode "Edith's Problem," the family discovers that Edith's recent irritability is due to "the change of life."[4] Husband Archie responds by being annoyed that she cannot go through this "in thirty seconds." Although intended to be humorous, Archie's inconvenience from Edith's situation takes precedent over what she is experiencing. A decade later, in *Golden Girls*, Blanche is depressed when she learns that she is not pregnant but is in fact going through menopause. Blanche's despair comes from not wanting to age. This episode, which aired in 1986, was titled "End of the Curse."[5] Sophia, from an earlier generation, explains that no one told her that women menstruate and no one told her that she would no longer have her period, either. Both of these sitcoms focus on the negative aspects of menopause, especially as it was experienced in the past. This is evidenced by terminology used such as "problem" and "curse," another term for menstruation.

More recent in the minds of today's midlife women is the popular *Menopause The Musical*, which premiered in 2001 in Orlando, Florida.[6] This highly popular production focuses on four women shopping for lingerie in Bloomingdale's department store. To that extent, it shapes menopause as a middle-class issue. The four characters, including one black woman, are the prototypes "Professional Woman," "Iowa Housewife," "Earth Mother," and "Soap Star." The musical pokes fun at women's experiences with hot flashes, irritability, weight gain, sagging breasts and changing body shape, poor eyesight, sexual frustration, night sweats, and worries about their own mothers. However, the intention is that women will find humor in their own situation and that it will normalize their experience.

Beyond this, there is very little discussion of menopause in popular media today, including print. Using content analysis on seven popular women's magazines meant to represent a range of interests, I discovered over the course of one year references to menopause in only one of those magazines.[7] *Good Housekeeping* included an average of one advertisement per month for the product Menopace™, a supplement including B6 to regulate hormone activity, vitamin D for bone health, and a soya extract for menopausal symptoms overall. All these magazines had photos of middle-aged and older women and included articles about their lives, but there was not one story about women's menopausal experiences or the positive aspects of menopause.

There are many more references to menopause on the internet. "Googling" the word "menopause" results in a number of sites that focus on the biophysiology of menopause, its symptoms, and how to treat them. Results include sites of highly reputable health providers such as the Mayo Clinic and organizations devoted solely to menopause, such as the North American Menopause Society (NAMS).[8] This latter site, which is maintained for both professionals and women, includes links to a page titled "Finding a Menopause Practitioner," a menopause guidebook, a sexual health module, information about hormone therapy, and a NAMS video series. The majority of sites include information on the top supplements to treat menopause and the most common symptoms of menopause.

The social media platform Facebook includes a number of private pages or groups devoted to discussion of menopause. The "Menopause Matters" private group includes 2,100 members and is geared toward a discussion of general issues and experiences. "Menopause and Mental Health Misery," with 315 members, focuses more on the impact of menopause on mental health. Rules included at the top of the page state, "No judging or bullying." A third discussion group on Facebook, "Approaching Menopause," includes 193 members and is geared toward women in their forties who have not yet gone through menopause.

There are many blogs devoted to menopause. One of the most popular ones, *Red Hot Mamas*, refers to "outsmarting menopause." One must join in order to take advantage of the opportunity to ask questions of "experts," access articles, and find out about talks and programs led by blogger Karen Giblin.[9] Other blogs, such as *Menopause Goddess*, include stories about other people's experiences and journeys that are relatable and inspiring and an opportunity to ask questions of one another.[10] Ellen Dolgen's blog, *Living in Perimenopause and Menopause*, includes links to a Hot Flash guide, Menopause Symptoms chart, Menopause Specialist Directory, and instruction manual called Perimenopause and Menopause 101.[11] Dolgen became an advocate after her own difficulties with menopause. She is an author, speaker, and awareness advocate. All these blogs are written in a chatty, girlfriend-to-girlfriend style. These are only three among a multitude of blogs.

Many of the examples of menopause in popular culture are oriented toward helping women to navigate their experience by providing information, other women to talk to, and even offering humor to buffer the difficulties of the situation. Social media also offers opportunities to purchase products that may or may not be effective in treating symptoms, thus capitalizing on women's needs and vulnerabilities. Although some providers of information take a balanced approach in recognizing both the positive and negative effects of being menopausal, others attempt to discount what can be a devastating experience. Most of the information is geared toward a purely biophysiological and medical construction of menopause.

THE ROLE OF MEDICINE

Our perception of menopause reflects not only popular culture but also women's changing roles in the United States as well as changing medical information. Medical historian Judith Houck chronicles how prevailing standards of femininity and social expectations of women, the results of both political and social events of the time, affected the medical community's views of menopause and its meaning in women's lives.[12] In the late nineteenth and early twentieth centuries, physicians saw menopause as a normal part of the life course that would pass. Not all women even lived to experience menopause, as the average life expectancy for women did not reach fifty-two years of age until 1901.[13] Physicians advised over-the-counter remedies as sufficient solutions for women's symptoms. Society in general saw menopause as a transition in women's social roles. Since they no longer provided a reproductive role, they were expected to maintain a public service by "mothering" others in the community through volunteer services.

It was not until the 1930s that hormone replacement therapy (HRT) became the remedy of choice for women experiencing menopausal symptoms. This period saw increasing pharmaceutical usage in general and the start of the insurance industry in the United States.[13,14,15] Though menopause itself was still seen as a natural transition, severe symptoms were believed to warrant medical intervention. However, menopause was only partially medicalized. Although women relied on a medical treatment, they learned about menopause through their friends rather than their physicians. Menopause was still seen as outside of standard medical discussion with a physician until it produced a significant medical problem. The fact that women sought HRT suggests that they saw their symptoms as requiring medical intervention. Typically, only privileged white women sought hormone therapy from their physicians.[16]

Some physicians, however, questioned the logic of medically treating menopause if it was indeed a "natural transition." Women's magazines urged their readers to take charge of their health care. Women were told that they would not notice the symptoms if they kept busy. They were told to control their symptoms so that they could still satisfy their husbands' sexual needs and to make sure that they continued to be attractive and take care of their appearance.[17]

The belief in the need to medicalize menopause was strengthened when Wilson and Wilson published an article in the *Journal of the American Geriatrics Society* claiming that menopause "defeminized" women. They argued that women should choose HRT to prevent the effects of aging and to maintain their femininity.[18] They did not mention any possible negative side effects of the medications. With this, the authors made clear the view shared by many at the time: that women's femininity and contribution to society were solely the result of their ability to bear children and to maintain their youthfulness. This article framed menopause as a deficiency "disease" and proposed a strictly medical model to address it.

Middle-class women and the popular media were quick to endorse this idea. For example, physician David Reuben wrote the following in his best seller *Everything You Always Wanted to Know about Sex*: "As estrogen is shut off, a woman comes as close as she can to being a man. . . . No longer a functional woman, these women live in a world of intersex. Having outlived their ovaries, they have outlived their usefulness as human beings."[19] Other popular sources also discussed the benefit of HRT to avoid menopause and keep women forever young. For example, the *Newsweek* (1964) article "No More Menopause"[20] and *Vogue* (1965) article "How to Live Young at Any Age"[21] espoused the benefits of added estrogen to prevent the loss of menstruation and the increase in weight gain, facial hair, and vaginal dryness that come with menopause. Other publications simultaneously minimized the negative health impacts of estrogen replacement. The *Ladies' Home Journal* (1965) article "The Truth About Female Hormones"[22] and *Cosmopolitan*'s "Oh What a Lovely Pill"[23] endorsed estrogen supplements as safe, with minimal side effects. Best sellers such as *Feminine Forever*[24] and *E.R.T.: The Pills to Keep Women Young*,[25] by

Wilson and Wilson in 1966 and Walsh in 1965 respectively, present menopause as an unwelcome change when women are at the mercy of their changing hormones. This was a major shift in the meaning of menopause, as it was no longer seen as a normal part of the life course without need for intervention. Interestingly, there was no recognition of the benefits of no longer being fertile and having no further pregnancies.

Many women supported this notion that women must liberate themselves from their biological destiny, that is, their changing hormones, in order to create social change. To them, it was the fluctuations in their hormones that needed to be controlled. The decrease of the very hormones that had limited them to motherhood did not matter. Later feminists would resist the belief that their hormones affect their behavior and health beyond that which can be addressed by naturopathy and exercise. They argued that it is patriarchy and a sexist society, not hormones, that control women. In addition, later evidence that HRT increases risk for certain cancers and other health problems fueled the feminist opposition to the medical model of menopause.[26]

Estrogen or Hormone Replacement Therapy and Risk of Breast Cancer

It was not until 2002 that findings from the Women's Health Initiative showed significant health impacts from hormone replacement therapy.[27] Started in 1991 by the National Institutes of Health (NIH) and National Institute of Heart, Lung, and Blood (NIHLB), the Women's Health Initiative was the largest study of women's health, with over 161,000 participants. Clinical trials that looked at the effect of estrogen alone and an estrogen and progestin combination found a 26 percent increase of breast cancer, particularly for those women on the combined pill for long periods of time. Researchers also found an increase in heart disease, stroke, and blood clots among previously healthy women. While the medical community was concerned about the possible side effects of hormone replacement since its onset, this was the first confirmed finding. Results of the study were quickly disseminated throughout society.

The SWHAN Study

The second major epidemiologic study of women's health during midlife, referred to as the Study of Women's Health across the Nation

(SWHAN), began with a baseline study of 3,302 women in 1996–1997 among seven research centers across the nation. It represented five major racial and ethnic groups. Results of this study showed a 50 percent decrease in breast cancer risk among women with vasomotor symptoms (VMS), also referred to as hot flashes. That is, hot flashes were found to be related to a decreased likelihood of developing breast cancer. Hot flashes are believed to be triggered by declining estrogen levels during menopause. However, breast cancer risk increases when and if estrogen levels are elevated. Thus, while hot flashes (or VMS) are experienced as among the worst symptoms of menopause, they may also lower susceptibility to breast cancer when not augmented by oral estrogen/progestin replacement.[28]

TREATMENT TODAY

Today, physicians are highly reluctant to prescribe hormone replacement therapy except in cases of debilitating symptoms.[29] Instead, physicians may prescribe selective serotonin reuptake inhibitors (SSRIs) such as Paxil™, serotonin-norepinephrine reuptake inhibitors (SNRIs) such as Venlafaxine™ Effexor™, Clonidine™ (otherwise prescribed for blood pressure), and Gabapentin™ (also used to treat nerve pain) for the symptoms of menopause when women present with severe symptoms of hot flashes. By preventing the reuptake of serotonin and norepinephrine, the body is able to regulate temperature better. Venlafaxine, also referred to as Effexor, is most commonly prescribed for menopausal symptoms.[30,31]

Physicians also suggest a healthy diet and regular exercise to treat the symptoms of menopause. A healthy diet is one that includes low-fat proteins, soy, vegetables, whole grains, limited fruit, and minimal amounts of alcohol and caffeine. Limiting alcohol minimizes unnecessary calories while controlling caffeine aids sleep. By providing a baseline of optimal health, women can better manage the ups and downs of menopause. Regular exercise improves sleep and produces proteins called neurotrophic or growth factors that cause nerve cells to grow and make new connections. The hippocampus, which controls mood and emotion, is usually smaller in depressed individuals. Long-term low-intensity exercise supports nerve growth in the hippocampus, improving nerve cell connections and relieving depression. High-intensity exercise also releases the feel-good proteins called endorphins that act similarly in the body as opiates.[32]

Physicians also suggest supplementing one's diet with vitamin B complex and vitamin E. Vitamin B helps to transform food into energy; assists the cardiovascular, immune, and nervous systems; works with the brain to produce serotonin and norepinephrine to assist mood and decrease irritability and produces melatonin to aid sleep. Vitamin E is taken for optimal cardiovascular health as heart disease is the number one cause of death in postmenopausal women.[33,34,35,36] Physicians further encourage a minimal supplement of vitamin D and calcium to decrease risk of osteoporosis.

Physicians may also prescribe bioidentical hormones that are synthesized from natural products, such as plants, to produce the identical structure of hormones as they occur in the body. It is their similar structure to our own hormones that makes them effective and (manufacturers argue) safe, in comparison to synthetic hormones found in HRT. The way they work is as follows. Hormones have a solid steroid base decorated with attachments similar to arms, legs, and tails. It is these attachments that turn the hormones into receptor molecules throughout the body, turning cellular behavior on and off. Bioidentical hormones used to treat menopause symptoms have the same molecular structure as the alpha estrogen receptors to which mammalian estrogen binds. It is mammalian estrogen that results in breast and genital tissue, for example.

Bioidentical hormones are found in vaginal rings, such as Estring™, and creams used to treat painful intercourse due to vaginal drying. Estring™ (trademark Pfizer), also known as an estradiol vaginal ring, releases a very low dose of estrogen (2 mg) into the vagina. Its advertisements suggest many possible side effects, but critics argue that it is no safer than HRT. Intrarosa Prasterone (Intrarosa™) is a steroid in cream form also used to treat dyspareunic, or painful, intercourse due to vaginal atrophy. This metabolite is also argued as less harmful than the original hormone, but critics question this.[37]

Women may also find their own solutions to menopausal symptoms, which can be used without a doctor's prescription. Although not determined to be as effective as estrogen replacement therapy, many women have turned to these estrogen mimickers. Phytoestrogens, found in soy and some herbs, are natural selective estrogen receptor modulators like bioidentical hormones that help your body adapt to its current hormone level. Phytoestrogens, however, bind to the beta estrogen receptors, the second type of estrogen receptors, allowing them to modulate the amount of estrogen and progesterone in the body. Their structure is a different shape than that of bioidentical hormones that bond to the alpha estrogen receptors. If estrogen is too low, phytoestrogens will have a tonifying and moisturizing effect on cells. If estrogen is too high, the phytoestrogen will exert a modulating effect to stabilize the cell and protect it from overstimulation. The herbs maca, pueraria mirifica, and black cohosh are believed to boost estrogen, while vitex is believed to boost progesterone.[38]

Supplements that contain more than one phytoestrogen can also be purchased online or in an equivalent health store. In one article in the *Herbalist Report*, researchers examined the ingredients in thirty-seven supplements found online for the existence of the top five phytoestrogens (soy, black cohosh, dong quai, ginseng, and red clover) and evidence that they relieved symptoms. The top supplement was EstroVite™, which contained all five phytoestrogens and, according to the *Herbalist Report*, was backed by evidence that it relieves symptoms. In addition, there is evidence that soy, taken in an equivalent of three servings per day, relieves the symptoms of menopause following twelve weeks of consumption.[39]

Although the effects are less known, some women have turned to Eastern practices to assist with menopause. There is evidence that mindfulness training allows women to handle better both hot flashes and night sweats.[40] In particular, it reduces the stress associated with hot flashes and night sweats and improves physical, psychosocial, and sexual functioning. Although the intensity of hot flashes did not differ between those who did and did not practice mindfulness training, those who did reported better sleep (i.e., less insomnia) and less anxiety and perceived stress. Mindfulness teaches its practitioners to be less reactive and more accepting of the thoughts that pass through their minds and that which is present in their lives. Practitioners are encouraged to avoid making judgments and allow things to be as they are. As a result, it improves women's resilience to the symptoms of menopause.[41]

Mindfulness training also better allows women to reflect on and reappraise their priorities, goals, and relationships. The attention monitoring aspect of mindfulness can allow people to be more readily aware of their thoughts and emotions, which can allow greater flexibility in cognitive reappraisal.[42] Mindfulness trains people to refrain from resisting uncomfortable and painful thoughts and to allow them to be without pushing them down into the subconscious. This allows practitioners a clearer view of what they may need to change in their lives and avoid the stress response that comes from resisting one's emotions.[43] Mindfulness also leads to changes in the brain structure, which is referred to as neuroplasticity. This is the ability of the brain to change throughout life rather than being fixed, as was previously thought. Mindfulness can allow its practitioners to overcome depression, anxiety, and some mental illnesses, particularly if it is combined with cognitive behavioral therapy. Neuroplasticity allows one to change overreactive patterns in the brain, such as negative thinking, and to create new neuron pathways.[44]

Mindfulness allows individuals to work better with negative experiences from their past because of the changes it causes in the brain. In a 2003 study, Richard Davidson, Jon Kabat-Zinn, and colleagues found that eight weeks of mindfulness training increased brain activity on the left side of the frontal region of the brain, the area of the brain that is associated with positive emotions. This activation occurred whether those practicing mindfulness were thinking and writing about a positive or a negative experience.[45] Others have also found that long-term meditation can actually change the physical structure of the brain.[46] Regions associated with attention, internal awareness, and sensory processing are thicker in long-term meditators than in a matched control group. Cortical thickening occurs with years of meditating, which offsets the usual thinning of the cortex that comes with aging. We learn to regulate our attention, such as learning where to place that attention, so that we can better regulate our emotions. Germer refers to this as "metacognition."[47] He argues that mindfulness gives one the ability to step back and witness one's thoughts and feelings rather than being overwhelmed by them and unaware of their source. Mindfulness thus gives us insight into the cause of our anger, frustration, or other difficult emotions and provides us the tools we need to investigate things we might want to change or reprioritize in our lives. It gives us insight into unresolved conflict in our lives as well. We learn how change is constant, how we create our own suffering when we resist change and emotion, and how we "cobble together a sense of self" that we need to protect. This helps us to tolerate pain better, knowing that it too will pass, and have the courage to address things we might want to alter in the future or new avenues we might wish to consider.

Being mindful alone is not enough to optimally create positive growth, however. Many researchers argue that the process of being mindful must also include acceptance of one's thoughts and emotions as well as self-compassion. Specifically, positive reappraisal of experiences can more readily occur if one is open to pleasant cues. Attention is broadened to include features beyond distress. Acceptance allows all experiences to arise and pass without further reactivity so that even stressful experiences are approached with a gentle curiosity and interest. This optimally stimulates positive growth for individuals, including menopausal women who are undergoing major changes in their lives.[48,49,50] Ongoing acceptance softens the distress that may otherwise encourage avoidant strategies that produce stagnation. "Attention monitoring and acceptance . . . retrain habitual patterns of observing and greeting the world in ways that translate to flexible and adaptive strategies for continued personal growth."[51] Leading psychologist Christopher Germer states, "Buddhist psychology and the science of mindfulness and acceptance-based psychotherapy prime the neocortex to take emotional discomfort 'under advisement' rather than slavishly try to eliminate it."[52]

In sum, there is an array of treatments that women may use for the symptoms of menopause. Lifestyle changes—for example, an increase in exercise and a nutritious diet including phytoestrogens, such as soy or certain herbs—are a useful beginning point. Bioidentical hormones and an SSRI or SNRI can also be used to modulate symptoms such as fluctuating body temperatures and vaginal dryness.[53] Mindfulness further helps women to manage the symptoms as well as to address unresolved emotional issues that may be magnified by changes to the brain. When these treatments do not work, or symptoms are disabling, physicians can also prescribe HRT in small amounts and for short periods of time, and therapists can help patients to work through difficult emotions. All these options work for both natural menopause and surgically or chemically induced menopause. This latter category usually causes more severe symptoms.[54]

A Three-Generation Case Study

This case study has the advantage of including three generations of women from one family. As such, it allows us to see how changing treatments and views of treatments affect each generation's social construction of menopause or the meaning that they attach to it and how they respond to the symptoms they experience.

The three women interviewed in this multigenerational family are all white and are all related by blood. Ruth is ninety-two years of age and lives alone in an apartment in city X. She has been widowed for more than ten years. Her daughter, Sandy, is seventy years of age and is recently retired. She and her husband also live in an apartment near Ruth. The two older generations have limited incomes, including their social security payments and pensions from the city of X. Sandy's daughter, Laura, is forty-eight years of age and going through menopause. She and her husband and two children live in the outskirts of the city in their own home. Both Laura and her husband have professional jobs and are involved in their two teenagers' lives. Together the three women provide a vivid example of how women's preferences for treatment and the meaning of menopause have changed over the generations.

Ruth was not prepared for menopause. For most of her adult life, with the exception of four pregnancies, she had experienced heavy bleeding and cramping during menstruation. She attributed this to "cysts growing inside of her," although she did not specify any further than that. It was because of this that Ruth was not surprised by the heavy bleeding that she experienced during perimenopause. As it grew worse, she decided to mention it to her regular primary care doctor. Ruth explained:

> I was bleeding a lot and not sleeping, so I went to my daughter's doctor at her insistence. I did not go to a ladies' doctor. I still don't. I just told him that my monthly had gotten a lot worse lately. It had always been bad, but now it was really bad. . . . I knew it was the right thing to mention it to the doctor, but you just did not talk about that sort of thing in those days. It was not polite conversation. . . . Now people talk about . . . well, everything. I guess it is for the better, but I just don't like it for myself.

Ruth's medical doctor told her that she might be going through menopause, although he did not explain what that term meant. Neither did Ruth ask him what it meant. She did later remember her mother telling her that someday she would not have her "monthly" anymore. None of her friends discussed menopause, though, and she did not have any sisters with whom she could discuss the topic. Her daughter did not mention it, although she might have known about it. Ruth explained:

> Well, he told me that I probably had menopause, but I really did not know what that meant. I did not want to tell him that though. . . . Then on the drive home I remembered my mother saying that I would not always have my period, and that made sense given what the doctor had said about how I would continue to have a heavy monthly before I eventually stopped and that it would be soon. . . . He told me he would give me something for it, but at that point I did not need anything.

Ruth would go on to have severe hot flashes, though, which prompted her to go back to her daughter's physician. She explained:

> I had to have my gall bladder out, and the nurse noticed my hot flashes. By then I had talked to my best friend . . . and daughter . . .

about what was happening, so I knew what it was. The nurse said that I should see my doctor about them because I had them often and there was lots that doctors could do about it. So when I went to see him again after my surgery, I told him about the hot flashes. He gave me a pill, which I took. I did not take it for very long though because the hot flashes went away soon after that. When I ran out of the pills I just did not go back.

When I asked Ruth if her doctor had given her estrogen pills, she stated that he probably had. This was also confirmed by her daughter. Sandy was not aware of how long her mother had taken the pills, although she did not think that it had been more than a few months. Ruth never did develop breast cancer or the other health problems associated with HRT, which may have been due to her short exposure.
Ruth added:

My daughter said some women got breast cancer from . . . the pills . . . and babies born without arms and legs from taking pills for morning sickness. I did not get breast cancer though and did not take those other pills, so I was lucky. I was lucky, and my family was lucky. . . . The more I think about it, I don't think I took the . . . the pills . . . for long, less than one year.

However, Ruth's daughter, Sandy, would tell me that Ruth had some emotional difficulty associated with menopause. According to Sandy, it was during this time that Ruth and her husband separated and divorced, although they would later move in together again. Sandy said:

It was like my mother just flipped her lid. She was convinced that my father was having an affair. She convinced herself. I really don't think he was, but I could not convince her of that. . . . I did convince her to see a psychiatrist at that time because she really seemed like she lost her mind, accusing the lady he worked with . . . of the two of them . . . and things like that. Her psychiatrist put her on Valium™ which she was on for the rest of her life. . . . We had to fight my mother to go there, but not to take the valium. My mother had this terrible fear of ending up on P6 [floor 6, the psychiatric ward of the hospital] . . . A couple of years later they got back together again, but they never remarried. . . . I think it scarred our family.

Sandy's first symptoms of menopause started around forty-eight years of age. She knew, as soon as they started, that she was beginning menopause.

She said, "Some of my friends were already having menopause, so I had seen them having hot flashes. Then I thought about how tired I had been and how irritable I was sometimes. So I knew."

Sandy, like her mother, did not see a gynecologist. She did, however, tell her primary care doctor that she was having hot flashes and, by then, missed periods. She explained:

> I told him just to make sure that things were like they were supposed to be. I suppose that I was just a little scared. . . . My mother had taken estrogen for a very short period, and I knew that there [were] some problems about cancer. I did not want to take any chances, so I did not ask [about estrogen]. I just said I wanted to make sure that everything was on track and okay. . . . I also bought a book and read that, which made me feel better. . . . I could talk to my friends, but I never would have talked to my mother about it. She would not have been helpful.

Sandy said that hot flashes were the worst part of menopause for her. She sought relief by going outside in the wintertime and standing in front of the air conditioner during the summer. She said, "That was when I insisted to my husband that we had to get an air conditioner for our bedroom. I did not care about any other part of the house as long as I could go in there for a relief. He understood that I was not kidding, and we went out and got the air conditioner that weekend." Sandy said that she probably yelled at her husband and kids more than she usually did during that time but that there were no real problems from it. She said, "My husband used to tell the kids when he saw me go out at winter that I had just gone out to be by myself and they should not bother me. They knew what was going on, at least my daughter did. My son must have known enough not to ask questions." Sandy also explained that her family was annoyed with her for keeping the heat so low all the time. She said, "I used to tell them that I was trying to save [money] on heat and they should wear layers. It didn't go over very well. If the kids put the heat up, I would put it down again."

Sandy's hot flashes lasted for approximately two years, but they were more than a nuisance for only about one year. Like her mother, Ruth, Sandy always had heavy bleeding during her period, and this did not worsen for her. Sandy described her menopause experience thus:

> I never really thought about it, but I guess I was lucky. Menopause was not too bad for me. I could handle the hot flashes okay, and I did

not lose my temper with my family any more than normal. . . . I did not have the [emotional] ups and downs that my mother did. . . . I am glad that I never did use the estrogen, because they later proved that it does cause breast cancer. I have had a number of friends with breast cancer. . . . I dreaded menopause, and it was about what I expected, but nothing more.

Laura, at forty-eight years of age, was experiencing hot flashes, insomnia, and erratic periods. Her perimenopausal experience started with erratic periods. It was not until she started having hot flashes that she realized that she was perimenopausal. She said:

> The hot flashes are borderline tolerable. I won't go on estrogen. I know that. They are hard to handle though. Sometimes at work, it just gets to be too much. I am a [dental] hygienist, and I have to wear a face mask and scrubs. I can't really peel any- thing off. Fortunately, our offices are air-conditioned. I don't know what I would do without that. . . . I cope by doing a sort of meditation. I focus on my breath; I lean into it. That is what I call it anyway. I don't try to fight it; I rec- ognize it for what it is at that moment. I concentrate on my breath and that the moment will pass, which it does. It is how I handled cramps, too . . . and problems with my kids. I concentrate on my breath and the moment . . . and acceptance for what is happening at that moment.

Laura said that she is also careful about her diet, avoiding caffeine and alcohol now that she is going through menopause. She works out on a step-per machine several times a week and attends a fitness class on the week-ends. Laura said that she has also added soy to her diet because she read that it reduces hot flashes, and she thinks it has to a small degree. Laura said that she might try acupuncture for the hot flashes if they worsen, but she hopes that she would not have to do that. Laura said that she has read several books about menopause and consulted a website that her gynecolo-gist recommended to her.

All three of the women said that they viewed menopause as a natural part of the life course. However, Ruth willingly accepted her doctor's pharmacological solution to her hot flashes without considering other alternatives or questioning her doctor. In contrast, Laura, the youngest generation, was certain that she would not use hormone replacement ther-apy and instead changed her lifestyle, with attention to diet and exercise, and used meditation to cope with her symptoms. Laura talked about her experience with more people than her mother and grandmother, especially her grandmother. Sandy, the middle generation, sought some information, but not as much as her daughter. Sandy was able to cope with her symptoms, but she did so by infringing on the comfort of other family members. In contrast, Laura's coping mechanism was more deliberate and controlled. Interestingly, it was Ruth who experienced more emotional difficulties with menopause, although she did not seem to recognize the relationship between the two. It was her daughter who raised the issue. Ruth's husband and daughter encouraged her to seek a medical solution, and Ruth did not question taking Valium, at least according to her daughter. Combined, this multigenerational family illustrates a transition from a medicalized view of menopause to a psychospiritual one that combines changes in lifestyle with Eastern practices and sometimes therapy as well.

All three generations of women saw menopause as an inconvenience. All had experienced difficult periods and were relieved to have them end (or expected to be ending soon, in Laura's case). Only Laura discussed some of the positive aspects of menopause. She said that she was glad to no longer be on birth control pills and was considering making some changes to her life now that her children were getting older. Laura thought that her marriage was stronger than it had been earlier in life when they were getting used to having children and were not as financially stable. In contrast, Laura's grandmother Ruth had divorced during menopause, possibly due to an associated depression at the time.

Meditation helped Laura to cope with hot flashes. It is also quite likely that it made her more aware of the mood swings that came with menopause, helping her to handle them more effectively. Laura also thought about the changes that she wished to make to her life now that her children were older, which may be attributed to mindfulness and, in part, to her meditation practice.

CONCLUSION

Throughout most of history, menopause has been seen as a normal part of the life course. This is because it occurs in all women as the result of a biologically induced change, a transition from being fertile to being infertile. However, it was medicalized, or assumed to be a medical condition that required pharmacological treatment, as early as the 1930s through the use of estrogen or HRT. In the 1930s, it was the remedy of choice for women with severe symptoms. By the 1960s, researchers Wilson and Wilson argued for HRT for all women to prevent the effects of aging and allow women to maintain their femininity.[55] Middle- and upper-class women endorsed this vision as they could afford it. Meanwhile, the media portrayed women as being at the mercy of their changing hormones, which they must control for the sake of their femininity.[56] It wasn't until 2002 that the results of the Women's Health Initiative showed a significantly greater incidence of breast cancer, heart disease, stroke, and blood clots in women who used combined estrogen and progestin; therefore, physicians began prescribing HRT solely for extreme cases.

With what does that leave women? Today, physicians prescribe HRT only for women with the most extreme cases of hot flashes, night sweats, and insomnia. Use of a combined estrogen and progestin pill would be given only in situations where women cannot function due to their symptoms, and alternatives have not been effective. Such intervention is more often used in nonnatural cases of menopause that are brought on by surgery or treatment that removes or harms a woman's ovaries. Whenever physicians prescribe hormone replacement, though, they prescribe the lowest possible dosage for the shortest possible period of time.

Physicians may be more likely to prescribe a selective serotonin reuptake inhibitor (SSRI) or serotonin and norepinephrine reuptake inhibitor (SNRI) for menopause symptoms. These medications are typically taken for depression and anxiety but can be used to stabilize body temperature fluctuations as well.[57,58] Most women, however, turn to spiritual/psychological and natural interventions though, as did Laura. As will be seen in the next chapter, some women take phytoestrogens like soy, black cohosh, or dong quai. Some also use bioidentical hormones for specific needs, such as salves and vaginal rings for vaginal dryness. Women have also turned to Eastern practices, such as mindfulness, meditation, yoga, and acupuncture, as well as exercise and nutrition to address menopausal symptoms, as did Laura. Proper nutrition includes a diet high in protein, fiber, and vegetables with minimal alcohol, caffeine, sugar, and processed foods.

Popular culture also affects our constructions of menopause. To the extent that popular culture reflects women's changing roles and medical information, the three are intertwined. Much of popular culture references the biophysiology of menopause and advertisements for treatment. Only more recently have we seen discussions of the positive gain that can come from menopause when a woman can take advantage of the opportunity to consider new options. Thus, it was the youngest member of the family discussed above, Laura, who discussed menopause in a more positive light than her mother and grandmother and who saw menopausal symptoms as something that she could change on her own with better nutrition, exercise, and meditation. Today menopause continues to be seen primarily as loss rather than a mix of loss and gain.

Chapters 6 and 7 will also discuss the value in using a combination of mindfulness and meditation to address some of the unresolved conflicts that bubble up during menopause. Physician Christiane Northrup argues that menopause puts a woman's private life and relationships under a microscope. This is caused by changes in the brain that enhance a woman's ability to recognize conflicts in their lives that have gone unresolved and to find solutions that they might not have seen clearly in the past. Northrup writes, "Our hormones are giving us the chance to see what we need to change in order to live honestly, joyfully, and fully."[59] I argue that we have gone from a society that medicalizes the treatment of menopause to one that embraces spiritual and psychological investigation and natural lifestyle changes.

THREE

The Range of Women's Experiences

This chapter looks at the range of experiences that characterize menopause. It is necessary for women to see how their experience fits in a range of circumstances to normalize what may feel very abnormal. Menopause is a transition not only to a new body and a new life stage, but in many cases, it is a transition to a new life or a new view on the world. How a woman gets there is as varied as the possible outcomes.

PERIMENOPAUSE

The term "perimenopause" means "around menopause." It refers to the time period in which a woman's body makes a natural transition to menopause. This is different from premenopause, which is the time period before perimenopause and menopause begin. During perimenopause, there are usually some signs or symptoms of progression toward menopause. A woman can determine if she is perimenopausal with an FSH test conducted by her gynecologist. Prior to menopause, the production of estrogen remains constant and may even increase a bit while progesterone falls. This imbalance in hormones is what makes the symptoms of menopause often worse during perimenopause. Levels of estrogen do not begin to wane until less than a year before the last menstrual period. As estrogen falls, the pituitary gland increases the production of the follicle-stimulating hormone (FSH) to rescue estrogen. During perimenopause, the FSH level begins to increase but it is not as high as it will be during menopause.[1] Some of the women studied asked their gynecologist to perform this test to see if some of the symptoms they were experiencing were the beginnings of menopause.

A few women had no perimenopausal experience. These women realized one day that they had not menstruated in months. They would go on never to menstruate again and to have no menopausal symptoms. This scenario, however, was not typical.

Typical perimenopausal symptoms included vaginal dryness, heavy bleeding during menstruation, irregular periods that lasted for shorter or longer lengths, periods that occurred more or less often, insomnia, hot flashes, night sweats, mood swings, and irritability. Cynthia stated:

> My periods were just excruciating. They would last practically the whole month. I might stop for two or three days, and then it would start up again. The blood was thick and black, and sometimes it just poured out of me. The cramps were worse than they had ever been...
> It never occurred to me that I could be starting menopause though. I always think of myself as younger than I am, so it just didn't dawn on me. When I finally realized [it], I went to the doctor to ask what could be done.

In contrast, Lauren's symptoms were related to her temperament.[2] She explained:

> I was a bitch on wheels, one hot mess. I drove like I was in a demolition derby. I was pulled over twice in one month for minor things, but I argued with the police officer like my life depended on it. . . . I also got in a couple of fender benders. . . . I hit a parked car in a parking lot and a rock, a boulder, at the end of a parking area. I had serious road rage. I yelled at a colleague at work, not that she did not deserve it. But I normally would have been able to keep my temper under control. . . . Then I did not know what was causing my rage. Now I think it was a combination of hormonal fluctuations and things from my past.

Hot flashes and night sweats were severe at perimenopause. Claire explained:

> I thought that maybe the kids were putting the heat up in the middle of the night. . . . I yelled at my youngest [for doing so], but she said that it wasn't her. . . . I would have to change my night gown two and

three times a night from night sweats. You could just wring it [the sweat] out. . . . I was complaining to my friend at the gym about the kids doing this, and she said, "Have you ever thought that you could be starting menopause?" It turned out she was right. I went to my gyn, and he took a blood test. He said I probably was getting ready for it and told me about some websites I could go to.

SYMPTOMS OF MENOPAUSE

The most common symptoms mentioned by the women included hot flashes, night sweats, vaginal dryness, low sex drive, mood swings, weight gain, and irritability. Less common symptoms included brittle hair and nails, less skin elasticity, aches and pains, and forgetfulness. A few of the women said that they experienced personality changes, depression, and psychological changes as well. Menopause was a time when some of the women reconsidered their career paths and relationships, made significant changes in their lives, or addressed unresolved issues from the past.

Hot flashes are a very common symptom of menopause. They can also be one of the most debilitating aspects of menopause. Most women said that they had three or four hot flashes per day, lasting anywhere from five to twenty minutes. Elyse, though, had approximately twenty hot flashes per day and woke up every twenty to twenty-five minutes at night because of night sweats before going on HRT. Women said that they could feel the hot flash start in their feet and legs and continue upward throughout their whole body. Their faces would become beet-red and flushed. Many women said that they learned to wear layers of clothing during menopause so that they could peel off outer layers during a hot flash. Other women would go outside during a hot flash, run cold water over their wrists, or place ice cubes on their necks.

Women with more severe hot flashes stated that it was the severity that led them to seek HRT. All but one of the women knew that HRT was linked with an increased risk of breast cancer. Those using HRT said that the increased risk of cancer was "worth it" because of just how debilitating the hot flashes were. Joy explained:

I had no choice but to use estrogen replacement. Yes, I knew that it had been found to cause cancer in some women, but I felt that I had no choice. I just couldn't go to work with hot flashes like that or with so little sleep. They [the hot flashes] were making me crazed. It is a wonder that I didn't lash out at someone.

In fact, Joy believed that the hot flashes and menopause in general were the cause of her divorce. She shared the following:

> That time in my life. . . . It makes me sad to have to say this, but I think that the hot flashes and all the menopause stuff played a big role in me getting divorced. I was just so angry all the time. My kids had left home; my husband and I, well, we had gone our own ways over the years. I think I would have at least tried to make it work, though, if I weren't dealing with the hot flashes and anger.

Night sweats and insomnia could be as common and debilitating as hot flashes. Women might have one or two night sweats per night, although some women had more. Elyse woke every twenty to twenty-five minutes during the night, often drenched in perspiration. Women explained that they would have to get out of bed and change their night clothes because they were so wet. Other women did not wake as often but might be awake for hours before falling back to sleep.

Women who did resort to HRT for hot flashes, night sweats, and insomnia continued to have symptoms, but they were no longer as constant or as severe as they were prior to the HRT. Elyse went from having twenty hot flashes per day to having two or three. Likewise, she now wakes up once or twice per night rather than every twenty to twenty-five minutes.

I asked Elyse and the other women how they reconciled taking HRT with the potential increased risk of cancer. All the women who took HRT said that it was necessary; they would otherwise have "gone out of [their] mind" from their menopausal symptoms. A few said that they felt defensive about their choice because they felt that they were sometimes judged for taking HRT, as if they were "weak." Judy said, "I would like to see a man try to go through a two-hour work meeting with two or three hot flashes and see how fast he went running to the doctor for relief." However, most of the women said that they reconciled the increased risk of cancer by taking as low a dose as their doctor suggested and planning to stop the medication as soon as their doctor recommended they do so. Elyse had been on HRT the longest. She explained:

> I started menopause around thirty-eight. I had my last child at thirty-seven, and I was having trouble with intercourse due to dryness. I knew that was common in menopause, so I went to my gynecologist. She put me on low-dose birth control pills that completely ended my periods. That was fine with me. I did not need my periods any more. . . . Then later I went for sleep difficulties and hot flashes. The

doctor prescribed low-dose hormones. Now I take a low-dose hormone replacement, Prempro™, three times a week. I have needed less and less [estrogen] over time because my body has needed less. . . . Every time I go in now, my doctor says, "Why don't we keep you on this for a little longer, but we will reduce the dosage a bit?" They [medical researchers and physicians] do not know the long-term effects, but I take such a low dose. . . . I really did not have any choice because the hot flashes were so bad . . . and frequent.

Vaginal dryness was another common symptom during perimenopause and menopause. Many of the women went to their gynecologists and were prescribed bioidentical hormones to treat the dryness. Bioidentical hormones come from natural products, such as plants, and have the identical structure of estrogen. As such, they act like estrogen in the body. Their effectiveness varied, with some women finding significant relief after trying a prescription and other women seeing no change at all. Women who found no relief from a bioidentical hormone cream or lotion said that they had to alter their sex lives somewhat in order to compensate for the pain during intercourse. This included changing positions during intercourse, but there was still some pain that was not there before menopause.

There were also emotional side effects from menopause. Most commonly, women said that they felt irritable and experienced mood swings during menopause. Similarly, others said that their emotions were "all over the board" during menopause. For example, Cynthia explained:

I just couldn't keep my emotions under control back then. It was like I became a different person. I was more feminine-like. I thought about adopting another child . . . even though our youngest was finishing up high school. I would start crying when I thought about some kids not having a home or family. Then I would be furious about what our president was doing . . . and I would start ranting and raving like a maniac. . . . I would yell at people in traffic. I think I felt like I was entitled [to yell] because I was older.

Also, I was so scattered. I would forget about what I was doing. One night I forgot about the chicken in the oven, and it came out dry and overcooked. I was gagging it was so dry. My husband was so sweet though and said, "Oh, I like it this way."

I stopped doing the things that I used to do, like getting a flu shot in the fall or getting my car inspected. I did not do Christmas cards that year . . . I just wasn't myself emotionally.

Some of the women sought help from a gynecologist because the mood swings and irritability were so extreme. They said that their physicians encouraged them to get more exercise and sleep, improve their diet and eat regularly, and to take vitamin B6. Vitamin B6 aids in the production of serotonin, which is a calming neurotransmitter that stabilizes mood. It is found in leafy, dark green vegetables as well as salmon, bananas, and poultry. Likewise, exercise causes the release of endorphins, neurotransmitters that interact with receptors in the cells found in regions of the brain controlling emotion. Their gynecologists, however, did not offer a prescription for an antidepressant.

More than a few women experienced depression during perimenopause or menopause. Most often they sought a therapist to discuss their concerns. A few of the women also sought assistance from a physician. Those who recognized that their depression could be linked to menopause discussed their depression with their gynecologist. It was often at this point or when hot flashes were extreme that gynecologists prescribed an SNRI or SSRI, neurotransmitters used to treat depression and stabilize body temperature. Use of the word "depression" during a doctor's appointment more often precipitated a prescription for antidepressants, whereas descriptions of mood swings and irritability did not. Stopping usage of antidepressants can be difficult, which leads physicians to prescribe them only in severe cases. SSRIs, including Celexa™, Lexapro™, Prozac™, Paxil™, and Zoloft™, are the most commonly used antidepressants. They prevent the uptake of serotonin in the brain, thus increasing the amount of serotonin, which stabilizes mood. In contrast, SNRIs are less commonly used to treat depression but rather are used to treat anxiety, obsessive-compulsive disorder, chronic pain (particularly nerve pain), and multiple menopausal symptoms. They act similarly to SSRIs but allow for the increase of both norepinephrine and serotonin. Norepinephrine is used for memory retention, alertness, and focusing attention. Typical SNRIs include Tramadol™, Venlafaxine™ (or Effexor), Duloxetine (Cymbalta™), and Sibutramine (Meridian™). Gynecologists most typically prescribe Venlafaxine™ for a myriad of menopausal symptoms.[3]

Very few women were prescribed an SSRI or SNRI for menopause. Women who did begin using an antidepressant were surprised to learn that it moderated their body temperature and decreased hot flashes and night sweats. Kathy explained:

> I couldn't believe it. I went in for the depression I was dealing with. I went to my gyn rather than my PCP because I like her better. She

said that it could be part of menopause and took a blood test. She said that I was probably going through menopause. I should have known. . . . So she prescribed Effexor. . . . It took about a month for it to work, but I noticed that I felt less like biting off someone's head. I did not notice it at first, though, but I was also having fewer night sweats and hot flashes. When I went back to see her, I told her, and she said that that was common. I was ecstatic. I wish that I had gone sooner. I could have prevented a couple of years of hot flashes.

Nina experienced even greater psychological changes during menopause. She underwent significant anxiety, panic attacks, and mania during menopause. Nina believed that the panic attacks were due to unresolved issues from a family member's death. During this time, Nina was seeing her regular primary care provider (PCP), a psychiatric nurse practitioner, a naturopath, an acupuncturist, and an endocrinologist. She reached the point where she was no longer able to function and had to take a three-week leave of absence from work to address her needs. Nina believed that the fluctuating hormones from menopause brought attention to or worsened abnormal levels of thyroid-stimulating hormones. Once an endocrinologist stabilized her thyroid, she began taking Effexor™ for her anxiety and panic attacks. Meanwhile, Nina saw an acupuncturist to "get her stabilized." It was Nina's son who suggested the use of an acupuncturist. Acupuncture is a traditional Chinese medicine used to balance the flow of energy, or chi, through the body. This is done by placing very tiny needles along the pathway or meridian points through which energy flows. Nina believed that rebalancing her energy flow also allowed her to get her panic attacks and mania under control. Nina also started seeing a therapist to address difficulties from her past. Nina said that she stayed on the Effexor™ for two years and saw a therapist for more than three years.

Nina's personality also changed during menopause. Her friends and family told her that she became much more paranoid that something would harm her or her family. She stopped planning as much as she always had and became more spontaneous. She said that she did not worry as much as she always had. Nina noticed that she was thinking more about the second half of her life and the implications of having a finite number of years left. She worried less about making mistakes and focused more on enjoying each day.

Most women began having menopausal or perimenopausal symptoms in their forties and early fifties. However, it was not uncommon for women to have menopausal symptoms as early as thirty-seven or thirty-eight years of age. Elyse first started having vaginal dryness at thirty-seven years old.

Others started having hot flashes at thirty-eight years of age. Thus, peri-menopausal symptoms typically begin between thirty-seven and fifty-two years of age. Menopausal symptoms lessen after not having a period for one year but may still continue at a lower level of intensity throughout life. Some of the women said that their mothers, who were in their early eighties, continued to have some hot flashes and wore layered clothing as a result.

USE OF PHYSICIANS

Not all women sought a physician's advice prior to or during menopause. African American and Latina women were much more likely to talk to their friends about their symptoms, if they sought any advice at all. Most women said that they mentioned symptoms during their annual physicals with a gynecologist or asked questions about their options for treatment at this time. However, those women who were experiencing very severe symptoms made a specific appointment with a gynecologist to discuss their options. It was at this time that their doctor sometimes took a blood test to measure levels of the FSH to test for menopause. This did not occur regularly, though.

Physicians typically suggested that women get more exercise and eat a healthy diet if they were having any menopausal symptoms. A few women remembered their doctor's advice to reduce caffeine and sugar during menopause and cut back on alcohol consumption. Others remembered physicians suggesting that they consume more soy, although some did not notice any difference in symptoms from doing so. As mentioned previously, a few physicians prescribed an antidepressant and/or therapy.

It is interesting to note that none of the women remembered physicians suggesting additional alternative treatments. For example, no one suggested meditation or mindfulness, which has been found to reduce stress and depression.[4,5,6,7] There is even evidence that it can help women to manage hot flashes better.[8] Physicians did not suggest any Eastern practices such as acupuncture, yoga, or massage to treat menopause. Physicians did suggest bioidentical hormones, especially the use of creams to treat vaginal dryness. None of the women had physicians who suggested use of supplements containing phytoestrogens, but a few did point out that soy may be effective in treating symptoms.

It was also rare for physicians to suggest HRT for their patients. Sallie had to have a hysterectomy due to ovarian cancer. She had hot flashes and insomnia even before the hysterectomy, but they worsened afterward. Sallie said that she was worried about HRT even before seeing her doctor because of a history of cancer and breast cancer in her family. When the hot flashes and insomnia worsened, her physician suggested an HRT patch. According to Sallie, the patch emits lower levels of estrogen than are usually found in a younger woman's body. For that reason, she is not worried about continuing to use the patch. Sallie said several times that she trusts the doctor who prescribed it. Elyse's gynecologist also suggested HRT when she was having hot flashes twenty to twenty-five times a day and not sleeping.

More women asked their physician about HRT when symptoms became uncomfortable. However, Sharon said that she demanded to be given estrogen/progestin at the very first signs of menopause. Her physician did give her a prescription for a low dosage of Premarin®, which she took for over three years. According to all the other women, physicians suggested that HRT be reserved and used only if symptoms became unbearable.

TREATMENTS WOMEN USED

What treatments did women then use? Most of the women said that they cut back on caffeine and alcohol and tried to eat a balanced diet. That included cutting back on sugar and fats as well as eating more protein and vegetables. Some of the women said that although that was their goal, their lifestyles often meant more fast food. Likewise, many of the women tried to get more exercise as they went through menopause, but as many said that they had never exercised regularly. Several women tried eating soy but had mixed levels of effectiveness.

Few women turned to Eastern practices for menopausal symptoms. Only four of the women used acupuncture to stabilize their body systems. A few others used meditation and mindfulness to manage menopause. However, several women used psychotherapy to address unresolved issues from the past. These last two topics will be discussed in Chapters 6 and 7.

Experience versus Expectation

Women by and large expected to have hot flashes, moodiness or mood swings, and night sweats with menopause. They pointed out, though, that they did not really know what that would be like until they experienced perimenopause. More often than not, women said that they did not realize how uncomfortable hot flashes and night sweats would be or how disruptive they would be to their lives. Neither did they realize how often hot flashes and night sweats would occur or how difficult it would be to get enough sleep.

Only women who experienced no symptoms or very few symptoms said that menopause was much easier than they expected it to be. Nicole said that she had some mood swings and two or three hot flashes a week, but nothing more. She found menopause to be easy because she had enough sleep to manage the few hot flashes. Maya and Kelly had no symptoms at all. They woke up one morning to realize that they had not had a period in months. They would go on never to have a period again or to have any associated symptoms.

It was more common for women to say that menopause was far worse than they expected it to be. Kathy explained:

> I thought it would be nice to not have my period any more. . . . I did not realize that it would throw my whole body into a frenzy. Hot flashes were a big deal. You can feel them coming all the way up through your body. Lack of a sex drive was also a problem. My periods were erratic, and there was much more cramping. I sweat like a pig and went from one to one hundred in a flash. . . . I went out a lot because I did better when we were out. I was a screaming lunatic . . . and irritable. The people in my life certainly noticed. Sleeping was a nightmare: falling asleep, staying asleep, getting back to sleep. I had a full-time job and two kids. Fortunately, I could keep my shit together at work, but I was a raving lunatic at home. I am surprised that the neighbors didn't call the police. Plus, the weight gain wasn't fun, either. I took St. John's Wort to help with my personality that had become a disorder. . . . I would tell people to be prepared [for menopause]. Whatever you have heard though, no matter how bad . . . it will be much worse than that.

Support Networks

The majority of the women sought some social support during menopause. Those women who did not seek support were more likely to be Latina. They said that they did not necessarily want to talk about menopause with other people, but they would talk to a female friend or their mother if they had wanted to discuss it. Carmen said:

I just don't think it is something that I want to talk about to other people. It is kind of private. . . . Who wants to know about that? Plus, I don't necessarily *want* people to know how old I am. . . . My mother knows that I am going through it, but we don't talk about it. I don't think it is something people want to talk about.

Not all Latina women chose to forgo social support during menopause. A few Latina women sought support from their female friends or sisters. Most often they said that they joked about going through menopause with their friends and sisters. Menopausal symptoms are often times associated with humor, particularly in the media. *Menopause The Musical* pokes fun at a variety of aspects of menopause: changes in sex drive, hot flashes, a frequent need to urinate, night sweats, and mood swings. Several of the women mentioned seeing this musical after menopause and finding it funny. They did not think they would have found it funny while they were going through menopause, though. Likewise, the women in this study found common ground with other women going through menopause by laughing about it. Valerie explained:

My girlfriends and I get together and joke about our hot flashes. We share stories about being absent-minded or distracted. Sometimes it's not funny, but mostly it is. We laugh . . . and we cry. One of my friends bought a blouse online. Then she saw an ad online and bought it again! She forgot that she had already bought it! She realized when both blouses arrived, days apart. . . . Another friend put her husband's dinner in the microwave and forgot all about it. She came down the stairs a little later and rummaged around the refrigerator for something to make for him for dinner. It wasn't until she was cooking *another* [her italics] dinner that she opened the microwave and saw the original dinner. It is just hard to stay focused now. . . . We laugh about our hot flashes, too. Like I said, it is easier to laugh than cry. Fewer worry lines under your eyes. We peel off our clothes and just take it in stride.

Women found it helpful to ask their female relatives and friends about their own menopause experiences. Questions centered around symptom management rather than the biology and physiology of menopause, about which all but one woman had basic information. They asked other women how long their symptoms lasted; what medications, vitamins, or other products they took for the symptoms; and what additional symptoms might occur down the line. Most typically women asked one another what they took (foods, supplements, medications, etc.) for menopause and what did or did not work. Kelsey explained:

> I asked around to find out what other people did. Then I went online too. I tried some of the things my friends did—soy, cutting down on alcohol, etc. None of my friends took estrogen, and I would not do that either. Online, I found some pills you can take and ordered them. . . . I think they helped. I had more energy, and my hot flashes seemed to come a little less often.

Women also asked their female friends and family if the symptoms they had already experienced, such as missed periods, could be precursors of menopause, in their friend or relative's opinion. Here they were asking their friends to compare their experiences. They found support in knowing that they could ask their friends for advice.

Women often asked their mothers about their own menopausal experiences prior to menopause. They typically wanted to know when their mothers had started menopause, what symptoms they had, and how long the symptoms lasted. They believed that their mother's experience might foreshadow their own experience.

Most of the women said that they found support from their gynecologist, particularly if they had a prior relationship with the person. Women depended on their gynecologists to tell them what treatments were most effective and safe. One woman said that her doctor did not go into much detail but sent her to several websites that were helpful. She found this to be supportive. Many women asked their gynecologists if it was safe for them to go off birth control when they first presented with symptoms of menopause. Women who went to a gynecologist during or just prior to menopause felt confident that their gynecologist would assist them in finding ways to manage their symptoms.

A number of women used the internet to learn more about menopause. Most used Google to verify that their symptoms were menopausal. Younger and more educated women went further though to seek out new information about menopause. Kelsey learned of the benefits of acupuncture for menopause through the internet. She also researched different supplements containing phytoestrogens and eventually ordered one for herself, which she believed had been helpful to her. Kristen used medical websites to learn more about treatment options and what to expect. Cynthia also learned of the benefits of mindfulness for managing symptoms of menopause from an article that she read online. It is important to point out, though, that these women also talked with their gynecologists and other women and sought support for menopause.

African American women were less likely to seek support or ask for assistance from a gynecologist as they went through menopause. They were concerned that a gynecologist might push them to have a hysterectomy or otherwise take advantage of them as patients. They pointed to prior studies that showed blacks being used as "guinea pigs" in experiments such as medical trials. They also pointed to similar situations they had heard about and negative interactions that people they knew had experienced with the medical community. These women did not believe that they had "lost out" on support from a gynecologist. This will be discussed in greater detail in Chapter 5.

Several of the women who had the most severe symptoms pointed to their husbands or wives as being essential support during menopause. As both their sexual partners and someone they lived with, it was important to them for their significant other to understand what was happening to them and comfort or encourage them when necessary. Kathy, for example, explained:

> I really needed my husband's understanding . . . and support. I was a raving lunatic, and I needed him to know it wasn't the real me and I wouldn't always be like that, or at least I hoped I wouldn't. . . . If I felt myself losing control, I would just say, "Okay, it's time for us to go out and get some fresh air," and he would know that I needed to get out. It seemed to help more than anything.

A few women mentioned friends who did not have support, which they found to be a failing on their friends' spouses' part. Several women also said that their own spouses sometimes blamed menopause for any annoyances that occurred. These women did not believe that their spouses were supportive. They did not appear to be critical of their husbands for this lack of support but thought it was just the way that men are. Toby explained:

> Every time I get down because of money or something the kids have done, my husband says, "It's the menopause talking." That makes me furious because it is not due to menopause. I really am upset about those things. . . . And it is like he just dismisses it. . . . That is how men are though. He said the same thing about PMS back in the day.

Surprise?!

A number of women were surprised when they found out that they were going through menopause. Cynthia had scheduled an appointment with a therapist because of depression. She said, "It just never even occurred to me that I could be experiencing menopause. It is kind of embarrassing because I think of myself as someone who is in tune with their own body. I just don't think of myself as being old enough to be menopausal, even though I am." Other women who were experiencing mood swings, night sweats, or irregular periods were also surprised. Rose said, "I have had irregular periods before, so I thought it could be due to fibroids again. I was pretty sure I wasn't pregnant. But menopause . . . I just had not thought of that."

Women who were experiencing hot flashes were not surprised that they had started menopause. Hot flashes are the most common symptom that women associate with menopause, and they are not associated with any other common medical condition. For that reason, Susan said:

> My first hot flash surprised the hell out of me. At first I did not know what it was. I thought, "Could I be getting a cold?" I looked around to see if anyone in the office was hot. Then I thought, "Oh, my God, that was a hot flash." I emailed my girlfriend who had gone through menopause, but I knew what it was even before I heard back from her.

NATURAL MENOPAUSE VERSUS SUDDEN AND EARLY MENOPAUSE

Natural menopause is the prolonged and gradual process of fluctuating hormonal levels that eventually ends with the last menstrual cycle. Women who go through a natural menopause no longer ovulate after menopause, but they still have ovaries that produce some estrogen. In natural menopause, the process usually begins in a woman's mid-to-late forties and ends in her fifties. However, some women experience menopause suddenly in their thirties (and sometimes even in their twenties) as a result of surgery or certain cancer treatments. This is referred to as "sudden and early menopause" and is defined as occurring before age forty.[9] Most of the experiences reported in this book refer to natural menopause, although there were a few women who reported either surgically induced menopause or treatment-induced menopause.

Surgically induced menopause occurs either when both ovaries are removed or when there is a full hysterectomy, which includes removal of the uterus and both ovaries. A full hysterectomy may be performed due to endometriosis,[10] ovarian cancer, estrogen receptor–positive breast cancer, and some other cancers such as cervical cancer that may spread. Typically, the ovaries are removed under these conditions to prevent the production of estrogen, which exacerbates the condition. The likelihood of surgically induced menopause is not common, but neither is it rare. One out of three women has a hysterectomy by age the age of fifty. Approximately half of these hysterectomies are performed on women under the age of forty-five. Further, 40 percent of these women have both ovaries removed. Injury to both ovaries can also cause sudden onset of menopause. Removal of both ovaries is referred to as bilateral oophorectomy.[11]

Women experiencing surgically induced menopause will typically wake from surgery with sudden menopausal symptoms. They are more likely to have severe vasomotor symptoms, that is, hot flashes and night sweats. In natural menopause, the ovaries will still produce some estrogen, but not so with bilateral oophorectomy. As a result, the condition increases the likelihood of heart disease, osteoporosis, and Parkinson's disease.[12]

The surgical removal of the uterus only, a simple hysterectomy, will not result in sudden menopause. However, it will hasten the start of natural menopause by at least 3.5 years. Ovaries require stimulation from prostaglandins, hormone-like substances produced by the uterus, in order to work properly. Without the uterus producing this substance, the ovaries will decrease production of estrogen much earlier. Removal of the uterus only may occur for extremely heavy periods, fibroids, and endometriosis that is contained to the outside of the uterus.[13]

Treatment-induced menopause usually occurs when chemotherapy, radiation therapy, and other drug-induced therapy for cancer damage the ovaries. The effect of chemotherapy usually occurs over several months rather than immediately. Damage to the ovaries, like the removal of the ovaries, will usually result in more severe menopausal symptoms compared to natural menopause. Sometimes the interruption to working ovaries is short term, however, and a woman's menstrual cycle returns to normal within four months. For most women, chemotherapy will result in the onset of permanent menopause.

Margaret: An Example of Surgically Induced Menopause

Margaret was a professional woman in her late fifties. Menopause began for her when she had a full medical hysterectomy at age thirty-three. This included the removal of the uterus as well as both ovaries. Margaret had always had erratic and very painful periods. She was in a committed lesbian relationship with an adopted son when she convinced her gynecologist that she would not regret a full hysterectomy. Margaret describes her experience thus:

> I had always had really bad periods. I tried to regulate them with birth control, but I would still get them every three weeks. I would go through a pad in five to ten minutes, and I even became anemic. They tried changing the dosage, but I [still] had horrific cramps. I did not dare to try to do things because I was always afraid that I would start bleeding. . . . Finally, I said to my doctor, "If you don't take it out, I am going to." He thought I would change my mind and want biological children. We already had [son's name] at that point. I told him I was in a lesbian relationship and that I did not want children. Finally he agreed to the hysterectomy.

That was the beginning of Margaret's menopausal experience. The surgery sent her spiraling into menopause. She had severe hot flashes that occurred multiple times per day and intense mood swings that she described as "huge, from real highs to real lows." In addition, Margaret experienced night sweats. She explained:

> If I had not had the wild raging mood swings, I could have coped with all else. We tried HRT. The mood swings were worse than they had been. I thought the HRT would at least help, but it made them worse. They tried regulating the dosage, but it didn't work. . . . It also caused endometrial tissue to develop. . . . I mentioned to my doctor that I was still having cramping and mood swings, and it felt like I was still getting my periods, so they did an ultrasound. That was when they found the endometrial tissue, and I had to have a second surgery to remove the endometrial tissue. [This surgery was laparoscopic.] I had tried HRT for one year, and it had made my symptoms worse and caused the endometrial tissue to develop. My mom had developed breast cancer by then, so I said no more HRT. . . . After the second surgery, all of the hot flashes and mood swings went away. I felt a great calm. I was so relieved.

Margaret was one of the women who found the most joy from menopause. She described it as a "freeing experience" and a "great joy to no longer have periods." She explained, "It is a liberating time for a woman to find out who you are. You can explore doing things you want to do." While the solution to the extremely painful periods led to equally difficult menopausal symptoms, the corrective changed Margaret's life for the better.

Sallie: Borderline Ovarian Cancer

Sallie's menopause came on quickly after a complete hysterectomy. After the surgery, she suffered from hot flashes, insomnia, weight gain, memory loss, acne, body aches, bunions, and hair breakage and loss. Sallie had suffered from acne throughout her life, however, birth control pills managed to keep it under control. Her acne returned with a vengeance in the absence of birth control pills. She made multiple trips to the dermatologist who prescribed topical and oral medications to get it under control. Decades prior, Sallie had a brush with ovarian cancer and had her left ovary and fallopian tube removed because of the possibility of a malignant tumor. Her doctor advocated that she have a complete hysterectomy when she was done having children because of this and also because of her mother having had rare fallopian tube cancer. She said, "[After the hysterectomy], I would wake up at night and be awake for two to three hours. I did not have mood swings or craziness, but my hair was falling out, and I had bad acne. I was getting the hot flashes four or more times a week."

Sallie's gynecologist recommended that she get a hormone replacement patch for the insomnia and hot flashes and prescribed a lubricant for vaginal dryness. Sallie said:

> I was so scared about what was going to happen. I was stressed about the hormone replacement because of the history of cancer in my family. My mom survived breast cancer but succumbed to complications after removal of a rare fallopian tube cancer. And I had a potentially cancerous tumor removed from my ovary. But my doctor pointed out that the patch would give me only a small percentage of what would be in my system anyway. . . . At first I wouldn't pursue it because of the risks . . . but I trust the doctor [who] recommended it. . . . The HRT patch has helped get the hot flashes under control, and melatonin is helping with the insomnia. . . . I guess it has been about a year now that I have had the patch. The gyn said it would be good for my bones and heart health, too.

Sallie was still experiencing some of the symptoms of menopause at the time of the study. She pointed out that throughout most of her adult life, she had had to supplement hormones for one reason or another. Sallie had to pursue in-vitro fertilization to become pregnant because half of her productive organs had been removed, and the remaining fallopian tube was blocked. This process involved injecting FSH and progesterone into her system, but it resulted in Sallie giving birth to two children.

Although Sallie saw menopause as a normal part of life for a woman, she still found it "depressing." She described menopause as "the perfect storm of the beginning of health problems." Now that Sallie is postmenopausal, she is still dealing with her hair falling out from hormonal changes, memory problems, acne, and weight gain. What seemed to bother Sallie the most was that she no longer felt youthful and that she had to permanently close the door to having more children in order to remain healthy.

A COMPARISON TO PREMENOPAUSE ATTITUDES AND EXPECTATIONS

A small group of women who had not yet started menopause were also interviewed about their expectations and attitudes toward menopause. In their early and midforties, these women were younger overall than those women who were experiencing menopause or who were postmenopausal. They were not necessarily younger than the women who had surgically induced menopause, however.

Women who had not yet started menopause tended to be vague in their descriptions of menopause. They knew that it referred to the cessation of having one's menstrual cycle and that a woman would no longer be able to become pregnant. However, they do not know any of the finer details, such as the fact that their periods would stop and start up again before stopping permanently. Nor did they know the definition of menopause, that is, going without one's period for a full year. Women expected that they would suddenly stop their periods at a definitive point. They were most aware of the symptom of hot flashes, but they were not aware of fluctuating hormonal changes related to menopause. Rarely did the women refer to changes in levels of estrogen, and none mentioned changes in levels of progesterone.

In comparison to women who had gone through menopause or were experiencing it, premenopausal women believed that menopause would have little to no effect on their lives. Although they believed that there would be a definitive point at which their periods would stop, they did not think that the symptoms would be impactful or that menopause would change their perspectives or priorities. They did anticipate feeling "old" when they reached menopause, though. In that regard, they believed that menopause would be a "turning point" in their lives. As a result, they said that they did not like to think about menopause. However, they were looking forward to no longer having a period. To them, "old" meant that they might not be as attractive as they were when they were younger, and they would start to get a thicker midsection. A few of the women said that they might have to take a few over-the-counter supplements for menopause, but they were not aware of what those supplements might be or for what they would need to take them. They saw menopause as a natural part of the life course, but they wished that they could avoid it all together.

Premenopausal women believed that there are natural remedies for menopausal symptoms that are as effective as HRT. They mentioned herbs that they heard were as effective as hormone replacement and were totally safe. They could not specify anything further, though, and were not familiar with the terms "phytoestrogens" or "bioidentical hormones." As was discussed in Chapter 2, there is some evidence that soy in particular can lessen menopausal symptoms, but there is no evidence of anything being as effective as hormone replacement therapy. Further still, some women continue to experience menopausal symptoms even with HRT.

One of the women also said that she was not going to allow hormones to affect her when she went through menopause. She may be one of the fortunate few who does not have difficulty with hot flashes or other symptoms due to hormonal imbalance. Most of the women who did experience difficult symptoms did not feel that it was within their power to prevent their symptoms. Neither did they believe that symptoms could be prevented by sheer willpower.

Premenopausal women had not taken any specific measures to prepare for menopause. One woman attended yoga classes but did not do so to prepare for menopause. Several exercised and watched their weight off and on but were not "rigid" about it. They did not anticipate making any such changes in their lives. They did, however, think that it might be a good idea to seek support, such as seeing a therapist. One woman explained, "I think it would be a good idea [seeing a therapist] because I have heard that sometimes women think they are losing their minds . . . going crazy. It would be good to have someone to keep you grounded and know that you are okay."

CONCLUSION

Each woman's menopausal experience is unique. Some will experience no symptoms at all, whereas others will have one or more of a vast range of symptoms. Their symptoms will vary in age at onset, frequency, intensity, and duration. Each woman will also construct her own support network based on her race, marital status, and availability of female friends and relatives. Not surprisingly, women tend to not seek support from male friends or colleagues, although they do seek support from their husbands. Women try different treatments and seek advice in different places. Some use the internet only to verify their symptoms, whereas others go deeper to look for new treatments. It is important for women to realize that there is such a vast range of experiences so that they do not feel alone or outside of the norm.

Although a number of women used HRT to treat their symptoms, they did not necessarily see menopause as being medicalized. They still stated that they saw menopause as a stage of life or natural part of getting older for women. It was the severity of their symptoms that led them to seek a medical solution. In fact, one of the women said, "It is both a life stage and a medical issue. Menopause happens because of the stage of life you are in, but it may be medical as well if you have severe symptoms." A number of women were hopeful that medicine would find a better treatment for menopause that was safer than HRT. As such, one could argue that there is some lag in women still medicalizing what was once solely a stage of the life course. However, we can also argue that, given that there is a medical treatment, it will continue to be seen as both a natural part of life and also a medical event, as the woman above stated.

More women are starting to see menopause as benefiting from spiritual/psychological or Eastern treatments as well. They use acupuncture, mindfulness, meditation, and yoga to treat some of the symptoms. They also use therapy to address some of the unresolved issues that come to light during this stage of the life course. These women are likely to be younger.

Premenopausal women in their forties were not as familiar with treatments as those who were perimenopausal. They were overly optimistic that menopausal symptoms could be treated with over-the-counter supplements. One woman even stated that she was not going to "allow" her hormones to affect her. They were not doing anything special to prepare for menopause and did not think that menopause would have a large impact in their lives. They did think that they might want to see a therapist if they felt like they were "losing [their] mind," which they knew women some-times felt was happening. In short, their expectations of what was going to happen were far different from the very difficult circumstances of many menopausal women.

These results support the argument that we are shifting somewhat from seeing menopause as a medical condition that needs to be treated with pharmacological solutions to seeing it as a natural part of the life course that can be treated with lifestyle changes and Eastern practices such as meditation. The women in this study all saw menopause as a natural part of a woman's life, but they were willing to turn to pharmacological means when they believed that they had no choice or, in a few cases, when they did not want to be inconvenienced by menopausal symptoms. Many women requested hormone replacement from their doctors but were denied. Those women who had not yet started menopause but who were in their forties believed that they would be able to treat their symptoms with over-the-counter supplements and, unlike previous generations, would be able to ignore their hormones. This suggests a significant change in expec-tations, although they are unlikely to be feasible. In the next chapter, we will look deeper into the social meaning of menopause.

FOUR

The Social Meaning of Menopause and Education

THE SOCIAL CONSTRUCTION AND MEANING OF MENOPAUSE: THE INFLUENCE OF CULTURE

Cultural Anthropologist Sally Dammery argues that culture has appropriated the meaning of menarche and menstruation. This has resulted in vastly different constructions of menstruation across groups and societies. However, one's social position, dependent on class, education, race, ethnicity, and marital status, affects not only the experience of menarche but also the occurrence of menopause. In addition to the social and cultural factors that shape both menstruation and menopause, the historical context and medical paradigms of the time period also affect the meaning of menopause.[1] This will be discussed in the following section.

Generational Differences

Our views of menopause have changed considerably since the second half of the twentieth century. This is evidenced in a study that examines the changes in women's experiences between those undergoing menopause in the 1960s to the 1980s and those who experienced it in the late 1990s and early 2000s.[2] The author compared (1) daughters born in the early to mid-1950s, many of today's baby boomers, to (2) their mothers born in the 1920s and 1930s. She found that the definition of menopause had shifted from a natural, developmental transition for the mothers to an increasingly medicalized view of menopause that emphasized biological deficits for the daughters. While the physical experiences of women were remarkably similar for the mother and daughter pairs, she found that they differed in:

- how they talked about menopause
- how they defined and treated it
- how willing they were to "accept" versus "fight" it

The author argues that menopause was socially reconstructed in the latter half of the twentieth century to be seen as an unpleasant marker of old age that requires medical attention.

Talking about Menopause

Mothers were not nearly as forthcoming in their discussions of menopause as their daughters were. One mother said, "Menopause just happened. We didn't do much about it or discuss it with others. It wasn't something that we, umm, worried about."[3] Referred to as "widow's plague," talk of menopause was not considered appropriate for public discourse. This may have been in part because menopause was thought to make women crazy and was even considered grounds for divorce. In contrast, the daughters talked about menopause with a variety of people, including colleagues, friends, physicians, and their husbands, with ease.

Defining Menopause

In addition, the mothers defined menopause as a developmental transition, which included self-evaluation and examination of one's priorities. They saw it as a life stage rather than a medical event or condition. One mother explained, "Menopause was a time when I shifted priorities and interests. It opened up possibilities. It was a soul-searching transition."[4] Margaret Mead referred to this experience and process as producing a "post-menopausal zest." In contrast, daughters saw it as a physiological process of an aging body. They saw menopause as a health problem or estrogen deficiency disease that needed to be treated and even cured with HRT.

Treating Menopause

Mothers did not seek treatment for menopause, as they saw it neither as a disease nor a problem. Daughters, in contrast, tended to seek medical treatment right away. Eleven out of thirteen of the daughters were taking HRT at the initial interview (just prior to 2011) to relieve menopausal symptoms. In contrast, those mothers taking estrogen were doing so for osteoporosis prevention or a postmenopausal hysterectomy. White women with higher educational levels and family incomes had significantly higher rates of HRT usage, perhaps because they were more likely to see a physician. Daughters knew that they should change their lifestyles to include a better diet, exercise, and strength training, but they preferred pharmaceutical intervention.

Acceptance. Both mothers and daughters saw menopause as a relief from menstruation and fear of pregnancy. Mothers accepted the changes that occurred to their bodies but daughters did not. In 1966, when many of the daughters were teenagers and formulating ideas about their own femininity, Robert Wilson, MD, and his wife wrote in their book, *Feminine Forever*, that the lack of estrogen at menopause leads to the "shriveling" of a woman's body, leaving her "old and decrepit."[5] Estrogen pills were encouraged so that women could be "feminine forever": youthful, resilient, moist, sexy, and desirable. One daughter said she would "use almost any means necessary to conceal, deny, or lessen the physical appearance of aging." For these women, it is the culture of youth that has dominated their self-perception.

For the daughters, then, the development of pharmaceuticals and the new medical definition of menopause gave rise to a significantly different experience of menopause. The media also played a significant role in changing the social meaning of menopause. In 2011, the internet had over eleven million sites referring to menopause.[6] Prime-time television had addressed menopause as early as 1972 in the popular sitcom *All in the Family*. These daughters also had much greater access to self-help books and magazines than the generations before them. They were the women who made *Menopause: The Silent Passage* by Gail Sheehy a groundbreaking best seller when it was originally published in 1991. Now in its sixth edition, it has remained the "bible" on menopause for successive generations of women.[7] The media also ran advertisements, driven by a "menopause industry," that gave women the perception of personal control over their individual menopause experience. Women were told that they could make their own menopause experience more comfortable and devoid of inconvenience by buying and using various companies' products.

Some women discontinued use of HRT following the confirmation in 2002 of the side effects of estrogen/progestin, including significantly increased risk of breast cancer and other medical conditions. However, the majority of the daughters (eleven out of thirteen) persisted in using HRT. These were the baby boomers who grew up with a medicalized view of menopause. They stated that the benefits outweighed any potential side effects. They also expected that the pharmaceutical industry would develop something better or that complementary and alternative medicine would discover a new approach to treating menopause. Nearly nine years after the 2002 study, one daughter said, "Until they come up with something better, I'll keep it [use of HRT] up."[8]

This study will look at how the current time period and the contemporary generation of women going through menopause, post–baby boomers, affects the treatment they pursue and the meaning that they give to menopause.

Other Cultures

The change of life is experienced differently depending on one's cultural assumptions about aging, femininity, and the societal role of older women.[9] In her book, *The Silent Passage: Menopause*, Gail Sheehy notes that the feminine role assumed by women in their fertile years is reversed after menopause in a large number of cultures.[10] In many societies, that loss of femininity is seen in a negative light. However, women may be given a greater degree of freedom after menopause than they were permitted in their reproductive years. Women no longer represent a "risk of pollution" from menstruation in societies where such women are sequestered. Nor does a society need to ensure that fertile women will not bear illegitimate children should an extramarital affair occur.[11]

Cultural assumptions affect the experience of menopause in many countries. A study of Tunisian and French women found that it is the degree of male domination in a society as well as social class that determines the different experiences of menopause.[12] The authors discovered that Tunisian working-class women (whether living in Tunisia or France) experienced menopause with intense symptoms and strong feelings of social degradation. Tunisia is a predominantly Muslim country where women have fewer rights and lower rates of literacy than their husbands and brothers. In contrast, Tunisian middle-class women in both countries experienced menopause as a severe decline in aesthetic and social value but had few symptoms. In France, however, women described menopause as involving few symptoms and little change in their social value. It is the greater comforts of middle-class women, then, that make the symptoms of menopause more bearable and less noticeable, but it is the low societal value placed on women in a male-dominated society that makes menopause an experience of social degradation. The loss of fertility and physical attractiveness decreases women's value in a male-dominated society such as Tunisia.

In some cultures, there is no concept of or word for various menopausal symptoms. For example, there is no word for "hot flashes" in Japanese. As such, Japanese women are less likely to see menopause as noteworthy. According to one study, 65 percent of Japanese women report menopause as uneventful.[13]

Chinese American women experience menopause differently from other American women.[14] Chinese Americans rarely report depression from menopause, and they do not see hot flashes as anything to be embarrassed about. As such, they are not as aware of hot flashes or as bothered by them. Even though women may experience the same symptoms, cultural interpretations and stigmas associated with the symptoms influence women's reporting of their intensity. Chinese women also have a different understanding of the development of menopause symptoms. Chinese women believe that the change in estrogen levels varies across women, and whether or not they develop "menopause syndrome" depends on how their bodies respond to that change. If the hormone level changes gradually, women will have few discomforts. If hormone levels change dramatically within a shorter time period, though, a woman will suffer more. Eventually, all women's bodies will get used to the new hormonal level, and all will be "fine."

Chinese American women tend to accept menopause and integrate it into their lives rather than try to change the menopausal condition. They understand menopause as the "order of nature" that cannot be altered by human power. Some have very positive attitudes about menopause and describe it as a life stage when women can take care of their "inner wants," which might have been suppressed in earlier life by family and career obligations. In contrast to white American women, Chinese women report that they use Chinese herbal medications to control any menopausal discomforts with enormous effectiveness, but they find that Western medicine sometimes does not work well. Gail Sheehy also points to the veneration of old age in China to explain the paucity of menopausal symptoms.[15]

At the Sixth International Congress on Menopause held in Bangkok in late 1990, researchers presented findings on the differences between women's experiences of menopause in Eastern versus Western countries. Like others, they found that women in Eastern countries report fewer and less severe symptoms of menopause than women in the West. Menopause in the West is cast primarily in hormonal terms. It is seen as a deficit of hormones, which must be replaced to rectify a medical malfunction. In contrast, in the East, menopause is less of a noteworthy event.[16] Likewise, they found that menopause results in significant social degradation in Eastern and Western societies where men dominate.

Gender Ideology

The dominant cultural story about menopause attributes women's behavior to hormonal changes. This may account for why some husbands discount women's menopausal emotional states. Instead of supporting their wives, they trivialize their experience.[17] Intimate partners reaffirm the dominant constructions of menopause when they encourage women to define their symptoms as problematic and seek medical treatment. Those women who report more positive experiences with menopause have partners who help in soothing their symptoms and encourage them to follow health regimens.[18]

Some women are particularly concerned about changes in their physical appearance and attractiveness after menopause. Based on norms that define women's beauty as exclusively youthful, they attempt to prevent and mask bodily changes in order to remain attractive, visibly feminine, and desirable in the eyes of men (if they are heterosexual). One study of sixty-one menopausal women in the Midwest found that all the single women and many of the married women worried about continuing to be attractive to men.[19] Single African American women were more convinced than single Euro American (white) women that menopause would make them less desirable to heterosexual men. Middle-class women had more options to control their weight, but others talked about ways they tried to control their unruly menopausal bodies. This was true regardless of race/ethnicity and class, suggesting the hegemony of gendered beauty ideals and their relationship to weight and youth. Those women who were most negative about menopause were concerned about their physical appearance. The author of the above study argues that menopausal meanings and experiences are determined more by the social constructions of gender than by actual body changes in menopause. In addition, women of all classes and ethnicities talked about how consideration of the effects of HRT on their weight played a role in their decision to use it or not. Finally, middle-class women were more likely to have tummy tucks, breast alterations, and face-lifts as a result of bodily transformations during menopause.[20]

Individual-Level Determinants

Individual demographic characteristics also affect women's experience of menopause. A study of 1,800 adult women in multiethnic Hilo, Hawaii, found that most women used positive terms such as "natural" to describe both menstruation (60.8 percent of women) and menopause (59.4 percent of women).[21] Postmenopausal women had more positive menstrual and menopausal attitudes than premenopausal women. They were able to look back more positively once the experience was over. Women who grew up outside of Hawaii also had more positive attitudes toward menopause. Having known a second culture may provide women with a broader per-spective through which to cope with the symptoms of menopause. Like-wise, higher education had a positive impact on anticipated menopause, suggesting educated women are more likely to believe that they can cope with menopause and that they will continue to have a role in society after menopause. Not surprisingly, negative attitudes toward menstruation and hot flashes decreased the likelihood of seeing menopause as a positive nat-ural life event.

Judy Strauss looked at the effect of one specific aspect of menopause, the loss of fertility, and how women adapt to it.[22,23] In a nationally repre-sentative study of over one thousand baby boomers born between 1946 and 1964, Strauss found that a number of factors help women adapt to menopause. Women with more roles as well older women have fewer con-cerns about the loss of fertility with menopause. Women with more roles, such as grandparent, caregiver, laborer outside of the home, and so on have more opportunities to balance their lives and find greater satisfaction in life after menopause. Likewise, older women are less likely than younger women to be in the midst of menopause or perimenopause when reactions to menopause tend to be more negative. Strauss also found that less edu-cated women have fewer concerns about the loss of fertility with meno-pause. She suggests that women with more exposure to information about menopause and the side effects of treatment may have greater concerns overall. In contrast, another study found that less educated women have higher risk of both physical and psychological symptoms of menopause.[24] Women with more financial security also have fewer concerns about the loss of fertility with menopause. Women with greater resources understand that their worth and value to society extend well beyond their reproductive ability, as was true of the French women in the study above.[25] Likewise, women who report fewer symptoms are less likely to be concerned about the effects of menopause on their health and level of attractiveness.

FINDINGS

Social Constructions of Menopause

The women in this study were asked, among other questions, their view of menopause, what menopause "looks like" to them, and how they would draw menopause. They associated menopause with many different meanings. Women typically provided more than one meaning of menopause.

The most common response from the women was that menopause was a "stage of life" or a "part of the life course." They described it as a "normal" part of life and a "natural thing" that occurs to women. Many said this in contrast to menopause being a medical condition. They tended to emphasize that because it was natural, they did not seek medications or prescription drugs. These women were more likely to say that they took vitamins, exercised, and maintained a healthy diet. A smaller number also added soy to the list of treatments for menopausal symptoms. They looked for natural solutions to a natural stage of life.

Some of the women, however, argued that instead of treating the symptoms of menopause, women should "let it happen the way that it is supposed to happen." They were asked what that meant to them. They said that women should not prevent the symptoms (hot flashes, mood swings, insomnia, and night sweats) from occurring because they allow menopause to progress and pass. Letting menopause happen the way it is supposed to, then, is learning to "live with the symptoms." One of these women added, "I just tried to be good-natured about it and not let the hot flashes get to me. I just laughed about it. It is nature, so don't buck it. . . . I tried not to lose my temper when I had mood swings."

Women who were using HRT associated menopause with being a stage of life, just like those who avoided pharmacological solutions. They pointed out, however, that menopause has biological changes, namely hormonal fluctuations, that need to be addressed. Elyse said that she sought HRT only when symptoms interfered with her life and made it impossible to function daily. In contrast, Priscilla said that she sought hormone replacement before she even started having symptoms, because she did not want to have to live with the symptoms. These women, then, did not see medication as contrary to something natural. Although a normal part of the life course, they also recognized that there were biological implications to menopause that required pharmaceutical interventions.

Women also associated menopause with no longer being able to have children or the end of an opportunity to reproduce. Many of the women said that this made them sad. They were not actively trying to get pregnant when menopause started, but it still was troublesome to them to know that they could not get pregnant. Cheryl, who had three daughters, said:

> I always hoped that I would have a son. It is not that I started meno-pause early, but I also had not been thinking about it. I had not given up the option of getting pregnant again and then it was too late. . . . It was the finality of it all and the fact that it wasn't my choice. Life just moved on.

A few of the women said that their reproductive systems had shut off. They said that not being able to have children, to no longer be fertile, meant that they were also "old." Similar to the responses of women from earlier studies, menopause was a loss of their youth and of their attractiveness.

Most of the women who associated menopause with no longer being able to have children saw this as a negative change in their lives. They were "sad" that they were no longer able to bear children. Others though said that no longer being able to have children was liberating. Claire, who was in her seventies, said:

> It was a relief to no longer worry about getting pregnant. We had . . . well, we had one child who we had not planned for. We could not afford to have another child. My husband is a typical red-blooded man, and I was relieved when I could finally enjoy our sex without getting pregnant.

Other women also associated menopause with freedom. Kelsey said that it was freeing to no longer have to worry about her period starting all of a sudden. Margaret said that it was freeing to no longer struggle with debilitating cramps and heavy bleeding. She said:

> I used to have to take a week off from work because my periods were so bad. I could not leave the bathroom. A couple of jobs I had to quit because I was taking so much time off. Motrin didn't even touch it [the pain]. I had a Mirena™ inserted to make my periods easier, but it did not help either. So I jumped for joy when menopause started and I was free from periods.

As importantly, women said that they associated menopause with being "free" to find out who they were and to explore the things they want to do with the rest of their lives. These women saw menopause as a time of joy. Shawna said:

> Now that I am through menopause, now that I don't have to stay home with my kids any more, I can think about going back to school. . . . My periods won't keep me from being able to attend classes. Also, now I don't have to worry about picking a career that will make a lot of money or that will make my parents happy. I am free to do what *I* [her emphasis] want. . . . Also, this is a freeing time to find out who I am. I have gone to a life coach to try to find out what I want to do. The coach used CBT [cognitive behavioral therapy] to help me figure out what I really want, but it also helped me to think about who I am and some of the problems, troubles that I have had with my family and that have held me back from being who I feel I am. I am tired of trying to always do the right thing and have the right kind of job. I need to just be me and do what is right for me.

Cynthia said that her personality actually changed during menopause. She explained:

> I used to be very shy, and now I am much, much more outgoing. I used to be more of a loner. I actually need to be around people now. Fortunately, my husband is okay with the new me. He says that my . . . sex drive is much stronger than it used to be . . . and that it makes him a little nervous. That just made me laugh. . . .

Cynthia was not sure what might have caused the change in her personality, but she speculated the following:

> I don't know if it is the change in hormones, but I think it might be. It might also be that I feel like at my age I have no reason to be reserved

or self-conscious anymore. I am at the top of my career. I have proven my worth at work, and I can support myself if I need to. So why be shy? . . . Also, I mind being alone now, and I have the self-confidence to be with people more. . . . I imagine that hormones have something to do with it too.

Nina believed that she also experienced psychological changes. She explained further that the change in her behavior may have been due to unresolved stresses from her past. Nina stated:

Yes, I was almost a different person. People told me about things that I said, and I couldn't believe it. I mean, I believed them of course, but it just wasn't me. I had a number of behavioral changes. I was absolutely certain that my husband was going to be killed in a car crash when he was on a trip. I was experiencing severe PTSD anxiety attacks. I refused to get on a plane. I had to leave work for two or three weeks. I just completely shut down and was paralyzed. . . . I had to see a therapist. There were things from the past that I had to deal with.

Karen also believed that her personality changed with menopause. This required that she also make some changes in her life. Karen explained:

When I went through menopause, I went from being someone who was afraid to someone who could stand on her own, be independent. After really looking at myself, I realized that I wanted more for myself; I was always *carrying* [her emphasis] my husband rather than vice versa. . . . I got a divorce. It was scary, but I did it. I would have been afraid to do it before menopause. I don't know what really made a difference, though.

For other women, menopause meant a time of confusion. Valerie said that she would draw menopause as "a person with a confused look who is saying, 'What is this?'" Kathy associated menopause with a person's whole body being in a frenzy. As a result of viewing menopause this way, she described her experience thus:

Menopause is very trying. It lasted much longer than I thought [four years]. People try to prepare you, but you have to live through it to understand. You give up your ability to have a child. All of sudden, I was old. It is erratic, hectic, personality change. You sweat like a pig. All of a sudden you go from one to one hundred. . . . Be prepared.

> Whatever you hear, no matter how bad, it will be more than that. I did not know that it would throw my whole body into a frenzy.

Valerie said that the instability that comes with menopause has resulted in some couples she knows having marital problems and divorcing as a result of menopause. She explained:

> I knew people whose marriages had broken up because of menopause. [My friend] was up and down, and her emotions were all over the board. She was a big hot mess, not stable like she had been. . . . They did not seek any help. The communication broke down. They would bicker all the time. My husband says that men need to be aware of what their wives are going through, the feelings of being in chaos. The women would not go for help, though. They tried to do it all themselves.

Similarly, some women attributed menopause to mean fluctuations in emotions and energy. Ellen said that she would draw menopause as a graph with spikes in energy levels and emotional ups and downs. Sharon was a very well-educated woman with several advanced degrees. She said that she "went running" to her gynecologist to insist on HRT before she even started having symptoms, despite being well aware of the increased risk of breast cancer and other diseases as a result of HRT. She said:

> I know, I know that estrogen replacement is known to be related to increased risk of breast cancer. I just don't want to have to deal with the mood swings and hot flashes. I have enough difficulties staying focused and in the present without my emotions being up and down because of raging hormones. I just needed something to smooth things out. I take a low level of estrogen and progesterone and will take it for only a little while.

In contrast, Ellen said that she tries to counteract the fluctuations in energy and emotions with natural methods. She said that she makes sure that she gets a good night's sleep and eats a healthy diet. Ellen believes that exercise also helps her to minimize fluctuations in energy and emotion. She takes vitamins, including calcium and vitamin D, to reduce the likelihood of osteoporosis, and she eats soy to minimize hot flashes.

Finally, many women associated menopause with getting older. Menopause meant being an "old woman." Elyse said:

> It is part of the aging process for women. . . . It is the body changes that occur when you are done with childbearing. . . . You have loose

skin tone, and your midsection gets thick. It is all part of getting older. [Hesitant] It is too bad that I associate it with that.

The association that Mara and her friends made between menopause and old age resulted in menopause being a very negative experience. Mara said:

It has just been horrible... I think of an old woman. All of a sudden you are old and decrepit. My girlfriends are even more negative. My friend, Maria, has always been good-natured, happy-go-lucky . . . but she has just tanked since menopause. She sees it as a low point in her life. . . . It changes us, how we feel about our bodies. It is sad because you are done having kids. I was done anyway. My youngest is in high school. But now I don't even have a choice about it. . . . Your body, it is not going to be like it used to. It is an emotional state too. You gain weight. You are cranky. A lot of my friends are taking antianxiety medications. They are so depressed getting older that it is making them anxious. It is so, so sad.

Sibyl added:

I am acutely aware that I am no longer a sexy young thing. In some ways that is a welcome change. . . . I don't want to have to go through starting all over again. But I miss being part of the girls. Knowing I am still sexy. . . . My middle is getting thicker, pear-shaped, like my mother and grandmother. [Laughs.] *God, like my mother and grandmother.* [Her emphasis.]

For many women, then, the association between menopause and old age resulted in their having a very negative view of menopause. These women tended to mention the physical aspects of menopause that they saw affecting their appearance negatively. They supported the belief that beauty equals youth and that older women, women who are postmenopausal, are no longer beautiful. Older women are still beautiful, but we are not aware of it because of a tendency for older women to try to look younger and a tendency in American society to leave older people out of the media.[26]

Education

A woman's cultural experience has a significant effect on the meaning that she associates with menopause and, therefore, the experience that she has. Women with lower levels of education were more likely to see menopause exclusively as a negative experience, not because of the symptoms that other women also mentioned, like hot flashes and night sweats, but because of the physical symptoms associated with age. For them, menopause meant becoming older, which they believed was confirmed by their thickening waists, looser skin tone, and inability to bear children. They associated beauty and femininity with fertility and youth. Like Wilson and Wilson, they believed that they had lost their femininity with menopause.[27,28] They did not necessarily adopt estrogen replacement to thwart menopause, but they did have to be medicated for anxiety due to their reaction to the loss of youth and fertility.

In contrast, better-educated women found joy and the opportunity to try new experiences and further explore their identities in menopause. More highly educated women noticed changes in their priorities and interests and were open to trying new lifestyles and careers. They embraced the positive aspects of menopause and did not dwell on the effects on their outward appearance.

Education also had some impact on the symptoms that women noted from menopause. Less-educated women were more concerned about their inability to have more children and the effect of menopause on their sexual appeal to men. This was true even though they had no intention of having more children and did not begin menopause until their late forties. Women with more education noted problematic symptoms such as hot flashes, mood swings, night sweats, and insomnia. However, they also noted more positive outcomes of menopause, such as being freer to try new things, having greater confidence, and being able to tackle issues from their past.

CONCLUSION

Women associate menopause with a vast array of concepts, from menopause meaning one is no longer able to have children to it being a joy and time of freedom. Most commonly, women associated menopause with a natural part of the life course and getting older. The meaning that they attached to menopause created significant differences in how they experienced menopause. Those women who associated menopause with no longer being able to have children felt sad about menopause. Those who associated it with vast fluctuations in their emotions and energy and who saw it as a time of confusion were more likely to discuss effects on their relationships and their female friends' relationships. They described it as being horrible and the worst time of their lives. In contrast, those women who associated menopause with freedom and joy experienced fewer symptoms and spoke more negatively about menstruation than menopause. They did not discuss physical symptoms but instead focused on opportunities in this new phase of life.

Less-educated women were more likely to associate menopause with aging and the physical characteristics of aging. Instead of discussing the wisdom that might come with being postmenopausal, they were concerned about the loss of their sex appeal to men and losing skin tone. They also were saddened by no longer being able to have children, even though they had no intention of becoming pregnant again. These women discussed their menopause experiences using the most negative tones.

Educational differences were more important than age differences in determining the meaning of menopause or the experience that resulted from that meaning. Women turned to HRT only when hot flashes and night sweats interfered with their daily functioning. The one exception was a highly educated woman who insisted on HRT because she was so distressed by the *potential* of mood swings or hot flashes. Many of the women did say, though, that their own mothers were reluctant to talk about menopause, some even to their own daughters. Perhaps these older women were more likely than their daughters to see menopause as a medical condition than as a natural part of the life course.

The degree to which women experience male dominance and entrenched gender ideology varies across subcultures in American society. Previous researchers found that women in male-dominated societies and those with stricter gender ideologies felt greater social degradation as a result of menopause. In this study, it was the less-educated women who felt that the loss of physical beauty and sexual appeal devalued them as postmenopausal women. This might result from less-educated women experiencing greater male domination. Although these women did not discuss severe hot flashes, night sweats, or mood swings, they viewed menopause as being the worst event in their lives.

The next chapter will look at the meaning that African American and Latina women attribute to menopause and the impact that it has on their menopausal experience. The African American subculture has a unique association with the medical community that has important implications for how its members understand and treat symptoms.

FIVE

Black and Latina Women and the Impact of Race

PREVIOUS RESEARCH

Race has a significant impact on the meaning and experience of menopause. A study by Dillaway and Byrnes found that African American and Latin American women, especially working-class women, see menopause in a positive light relative to white women.[1] They argue that the differences in experience, symptoms, and the meaning of menopause are created by dominant ideologies and the social constructions of race and class that promote unequal treatment of women, especially women of color. This greater unequal treatment has resulted in black women having a more *positive* view of menopause. They wish to differentiate themselves from their white counterparts, whom they see as unable to cope with discomforts such as menopause. Likewise, older black women serve as the matriarch of the family, which is less common in white families. As such, menopause does not have the denigrating effect for black women that it does for white women.

African American women and those in their social circles are distrustful of physicians and the medical community in general. Despite a greater risk of fibroids, which would suggest they might see physicians more often, African American women distrust physicians, especially gynecologists. This distrust can be traced back to the father of gynecology, Dr. James Marion Sims, who lived from 1813 through 1883. Sims paved the way for gynecology with inventions such as the Sims' speculum and the

Sims' position. However, he is also known for having advanced the field of surgery by practicing on enslaved black women without anesthesia. It should be noted that both anesthesia and ether were available at the time. Prior to Sims, there was no technique to repair vesicovaginal fistula, a severe complication of obstructed childbirth where a woman's bladder, cervix, and vagina are trapped between the fetal skull and pelvis, cutting off blood flow and leading to tissue death in the area. Eventually a hole develops in the area, leading to severe incontinence for which there is no treatment. Dr. Sims asked local slave owners in Montgomery, Alabama, to bring him slaves with fistula. Twelve slaves were brought by their owners. Sims performed surgery on all of them (and many of them several times) before developing a repair method using silver-wire sutures. Although Sims and his proponents argued that the slaves "begged" to be treated, they were essentially treated as guinea pigs. One slave required thirteen experimental surgeries before the vesicovaginal fistula was repaired.[2,3,4]

According to Dillaway and Byrnes, black women are more distrustful of the medical community for more recent egregious treatment as well. They and their mothers cite unnecessary hysterectomies from the 1970s and earlier, resulting in higher rates of sterilization for black women. They were also distrustful of physicians "padding their bills." As a result, African American women are more protective about the right to keep their reproductive organs and less likely to encourage one another to seek physicians' treatment for any symptoms. In contrast, white women made comments in the study about how hard it was for them to get an elective hysterectomy when they "just want[ed] to be done with it all."[5]

Black women see menopause in a more positive light for other reasons as well. In this same study, one woman said that blacks do not stress out about the same things as white women. She said that they are more likely to accept menopause, whereas some of the white women she knew had a "breakdown." She believed that black women have more important problems that required their time and energy. African Americans thought that white women concentrate too much on frustrating symptoms and worry about aspects of menopause that are trivial or unimportant. White women can complain to medical authorities about symptoms because they do not have to worry about racist repercussions, such as unnecessary hysterectomies. The authors point out that white, middle-class women have more access to medical information about menopause and its symptoms, which encourages their negativity.[6]

African American women said that they did not want to be like white women. In doing so, they assumed that all white women have the same standard reaction to menopause, which is not true. All individuals tend to identify with their socially defined category and see others as what they are not. Black women do not really know how white women react to menopause, but they are creating and reproducing a social "other." White women, in contrast, assume that women of other racial/ethnic categories have a menopause experience similar to their own. As such, they are endorsing the dominance of their whiteness. African American and Latina women are also less likely to talk to men about menopause than white women. They discuss it only with other women of their race, including their mothers. They do not see it as an appropriate "public" topic.[7]

Those African American women who did seek a physician's help were more likely to recount problems with physicians than white women. They believed that their physicians dismissed their concerns. As a result, African American women are more likely to rely on support from friends and family with menopause than the medical community.[8] In addition, black women are more likely to be steered toward a hysterectomy by their physician when they report symptoms of fibroids, for which they tend to have higher rates than white women. In contrast, the medical community counsels white women to wait for menopause to end, at which time fibroids will shrink due to lack of estrogen. As such, black women tend to be more suspicious of physicians and more likely to protect their reproductive organs.[9]

Race also impacts symptomology. Whites are more likely than any other race or ethnicity to report psychologic distress during menopause.[10] For all women, psychological distress was highest during early perimenopause (28.9 percent) and lowest in premenopause (20.9 percent) and postmenopause (22 percent).[11] Women experiencing psychological distress may wish to seek therapy or meditation and mindfulness for this distress, which is discussed in Chapter 6.

Gail Sheehy, while writing her seminal book *The Silent Passage: Menopause*, spoke with over one hundred women from diverse racial and ethnic backgrounds.[12] She argues that women who experience an increase in postmenopausal status and self-esteem are those who will (or will continue to) perform roles that require intellect, judgment, creativity, and spiritual strength. As a result, she found that African American women are more likely to pass through menopause with no psychological problems in comparison to white women. She argues that this is due to the dominance of black grandmothers in maintaining the extended family. In contrast, women who judge their worth on looks and sex appeal feel lower status after menopause and may therefore have more negative views of menopause. Interestingly, it is middle-class white women who are most likely to experience depression in this stage of life. Perhaps it is the knowledge that they will not have more children or that their children are leaving the nest that causes the onset of depression. For many of these women, child-rearing is a primary component of their self-worth.

Another cause of concern for white women is the assumed decrease in attractiveness associated with menopause. Prior to understanding the dangers of HRT, the factor most highly correlated with using HRT was concern for attractiveness among white women of higher socioeconomic status.[13] In addition, attitudes about menopause were a more influential determinant of using HRT than either physical or psychological symptoms.[14] As such, one would be more likely to expect white women to continue using HRT than black women.

BLACK WOMEN AND MENOPAUSE

Consistent with the findings of Dillaway and Byrnes, many of the women in this study did not seek a physician's advice while undergoing perimenopause and menopause.[15] These women consistently stated that they were uncomfortable or distrustful of physicians. Beverly explained:

> I don't go to the doctor's [office] if I can possibly help it. I just don't trust them. They say one thing and do another. . . . I have heard about experiments that were done on blacks like me. How can I be sure that they are not doing that and just not telling me . . . ? Plus, they find things that are not necessarily bothering you, but they go tinkering in there, and *then you are stuck* [her emphasis]. . . . You are better off without doctors if you can help it. . . . My mama, she never went to a doctor, and she came through menopause just fine. . . . It is natural . . . the way God made women. He did not intend for women to go on having babies forever. A cold cloth on your neck . . . that is all you need.

For Beverly, then, it was not necessary to go to a doctor for menopause because it is a natural part of the life course, and doctors are therefore not needed. Beverly was also suspicious of physicians and believed that they may find things that they think are wrong that are actually not problematic. Beverly was also willing to rely on what her own mother did for menopause, and she did not look to medicine to provide an improved solution to menopause the way that white women tended to do.

Ruth was also suspicious of physicians and unwilling to see one despite frequent, intense hot flashes. Ruth was also unwilling to see a physician earlier in life when she was suffering from endometriosis.[16] She explained:

> I have read about what happened to that woman, Henrietta [Lacks].[17] The doctors never told her that she had cancer, and they never paid her for using her body. Doctors would never treat whites that way. . . . Even before I read that book, I knew from my neighborhood about black women who were given a hysterectomy without their permission. They were trying to get rid of blacks, to end the race. . . . And then there were all of those experiments performed on blacks, Tuskegee and the like. They let black men have malaria without giving them anything for it. They never did that to whites. You never hear about whites being experimented on without their permission. . . . I had endometriosis when I was younger. It was very, very painful every period. They wanted to operate on me, but I wouldn't let them. I didn't have insurance back then, but that was just one aspect. I did not want a doctor going in there and taking out more than I gave him permission to do. Doctors will do that, you know, if you are black anyway. So I lived with the endometriosis until I found a black female doctor. . . . I don't have her for a doctor anymore because I moved. Maybe I would go to her again, though.

Women who were suspicious of physicians pointed to the fact that their own mothers had gone through menopause without a physician's assistance. No black women they knew had gone to a physician for menopausal symptoms although they knew of some white women who did see a physician for menopause. As they said, "Black women just don't do that." Thus it is part of the African American culture not to see assistance from a physician for menopause.

A few of the African American women said that they did see a gynecologist during perimenopause. Nicole, who saw a gynecologist regularly for uterine fibroids, explained:

> I was already seeing a gyn for fibroids when I went through menopause. I have had fibroids my entire adult life, starting in college. I have had to have more ultrasounds than I can count. So, I was just

holding on . . . hoping that the fibroids would shrink enough with menopause, which is supposed to happen with menopause, so that I would not have to have them removed. . . . So I saw my gyn regularly to check the size of the fibroids. . . . My periods got so bad before menopause started [perimenopause]. I was in so much pain, and my periods went on for almost the whole month with heavy bleeding. I told her that I did not think I was going to make it to menopause, with the fibroids that is. But she got me through it.

Likewise, Yvonne explained:

Yeah, I went to the doctor for the night sweats and hot flashes. None of my relatives and friends did, went to the doctor, but the white women I worked with did. She just told me that the only thing she could do would be to put me on an anti-depressant, and I did not want that, so I just lived with the hot flashes.

Interestingly, Yvonne's gynecologist did not mention the possibility of using HRT (according to Yvonne). Perhaps this physician did not bring up the option with any of her patients.

Consistent with the findings of Dillaway and Byrnes, black women reported fewer symptoms of menopause than white women.[18] White women typically mentioned hot flashes, night sweats, mood swings, insomnia, vaginal dryness, and sometimes psychological concerns or a need to reevaluate their lives. Black women sometimes mentioned hot flashes and night sweats, but they did not emphasize frequency or intensity. Only Yvonne said that the hot flashes brought her to a doctor's office. Instead, they downplayed the disruption to their lives relative to other concerns. Ruth explained:

The endometriosis was much worse than any old hot flashes. They were nothing. My momma cleaned offices and worked in a laundry. I wasn't going to complain about hot flashes when I thought about the arthritis she had and the aching legs that I would massage when I was a girl. . . . My dad used to pave roads in Alabama. . . . How could I complain about my life?

Other black women also referred to menopausal symptoms as being "no big deal."

Black women responded to what menopausal symptoms they did have with treatments they heard of from other black women. They referred to running their wrists under cold water, placing cold towels on their necks, and stepping out into the cold during winter to bring down their body temperatures. As such, they adapted to menopause. This was evidenced by the fact that they were less aware than white women of "false starts" when they had gone for months without menstruating but then had a period. For them, getting through perimenopause and menopause was not as great of a concern as it was for white women.

The gender ideology of the black culture also played a role in how women experienced menopause. Menopause was a less traumatic experience for black women because of the prominence of the black matriarch. Older black women are seen as sources of power in the family and are highly respected. Black men play a less central role in the family relative to white men because of higher rates of incarceration and deaths of despair and violence. Yvonne explained:

> Getting older isn't as big a deal for black women. We are just lucky that we *got* [her emphasis] to this age. We take care of our older folk, so you don't have to worry about getting older. Plus, we respect our elders. The grandmother is the most respected member of the family and community. She usually works and brings home a steady paycheck. She tries to keep her grandkids on the straight and narrow. . . . Usually she is highly involved in bringing up those grandkids, too. No, getting older isn't a bad thing for black women. They lead the family and the community. . . . And they run the church, too.

Thus, the powerful role that older black women have played for generations makes menopause less of a bad thing for black women. As a result, they are less likely to dwell on symptoms or dread its arrival.

Women's body image is also different in African American culture than Euro-American culture. Black women tend to be heavier than white women. Being heavier is not an anomaly at any age. As a result, there is less to dread from menopause. White women were continuing to use HRT, whereas none of the black women used it in this study. As was suggested by the literature, this may be due to white women's greater concern about the impact of menopause on their level of attractiveness. Black women are also less dependent on black men in a myriad of ways. Instead, older black women find worth in their family and community roles and in the black church.

LATINA WOMEN

The Latina women in this study responded with two disparate social constructions of menopause. Some of the Latina women provided the most assertive responses in this study. They saw menopause as a nuisance that needed to be combated. Michelle, for example, stated, "I am a forty-six-year-old woman, and I am not gonna let menopause get me down. . . . I have been through a lot in my life, and hot flashes are just a drop in the bucket."

Michelle was not aware that menopause was due to an imbalance in hormones, but she was aware that it had to do with aging and no longer being able to have children. She added:

> I don't let it bother me that I am getting older. It is just a number. I ain't crying on about not having more kids because I got my kids. . . . Some of my kids aren't even my kids. Life goes on, but I don't let hot flashes bother me. I take off my sweatshirt, my sweater, and spray cold water on my face. Sometimes I just go take a cold shower. . . . You have to be tough in this life and not be a victim to everything around you.

Another Latina woman explained, "I have people depending on me: my family, my grandbabies. You just have to be strong, the strong one." When asked what advice they would give to others, these women said to "be strong," "don't let the hot flashes get you down," and "get right back up." Interestingly, they also said that the symptoms of menopause were worse than they thought they would be, so their reactions were not due to having no or minimal symptoms. They thought that they had other priorities to focus on in life and that "conquering" menopause was the right response.

The second group of Latina women took a less combative approach to menopause. Several of these women pointed out that because it is a natural part of the life course, women "should just let it happen as it is supposed to." They were not trying to find a treatment to stop or lessen the symptoms. They saw no reason to fight a normal process but instead believed that women should allow it to occur naturally. It is important to note that none of these women had surgically induced or treatment-induced menopause, which typically results in more severe symptoms. While some described very bothersome hot flashes and night sweats that made it difficult to function optimally, they still chose not to see a doctor or request a pharmacological intervention.

When asked what they would suggest to other women going through menopause, they typically suggested behaviors related to a healthy lifestyle. One Latina woman recommended drinking plenty of water. Another suggested eating a healthy diet and exercising. One woman did not know what hormone replacement therapy was. Latina women also tended not to talk to others about menopause, particularly to men, including husbands and other male family members. Maria said:

> No, I don't talk to my husband about that. He doesn't want to hear about talk like that. What could he do about it anyway? . . . He might have some idea of it. He was probably still living at home when his mother was going through it. Men don't want to hear about that, though.

This second group of Latina women was also less likely to discuss their symptoms with friends and family. They talked with a much smaller group of confidantes, such as sisters or close friends. As such, they had a much smaller support system, if they had one at all. They also had less information available to them. Fewer Latina women used the internet to find information or talked with a physician, in addition to knowing fewer women with information.

Latin women saw menopause as a natural occurrence, but still they were embarrassed by being menopausal. These women were tight-lipped about their circumstances, especially compared to the first group of Latina women, who were quite vocal about their thoughts on the subject. This second group was very concerned about weight gain from menopause and getting older. They talked about the changes to their bodies, such as having a thicker midsection or being more pear-shaped. Perhaps they did not want to draw attention to their aging and heavier bodies.

Several of the women in this second group also mentioned other people being angry with them for some of their symptoms. Ruth, for example, said that her daughter was often very angry with her for being forgetful. Maria's husband grew angry with her when she opened the windows or turned down the heat because of her hot flashes. Likewise, Rose's son would walk out of the house when she became "too weepy."

A few of the Latina women discussed menopause in relation to menstruation and pregnancy. For them, the three conditions were all related to one another and to being female in general. For example, Carmen said:

> I am going through menopause because I used to have periods. And I used to have periods so that I could have babies. . . . Women, we drew the short straw in life. It is the price that we pay. . . . I tell my daughter that it's okay . . . having periods. That someday she will miss having periods just like someday she will miss being pregnant. You can't have one without the other. You go from one to the other.

Likewise, Theresa said that menopause means being female. She said that it means being a mother and a wife, but eventually the female body needs to rest. She added:

Being a mother means suffering for your children, worrying about them. Their problems get bigger as they get older. You are constantly worried about where they might be and whether or not they are safe. . . . It is the same thing. Menopause is worse than having your period in some ways . . . the hot flashes, flying off the handle, not sleeping . . . but it is all part of having children, and you love your children. Family is what it is all about, but it is hard being a mother.

This second group's reaction to menopause may be due, in part, to the machismo Latin culture where men dominate. Women were concerned that they were losing their attractiveness and did not want to call attention to it. They also had no respected roles to look forward to in old age compared to the matriarchal black women. Neither did they seem to have a strong support system like black women. Therefore, Latin women's social construction of menopause was much more negative than that of black women.

The Social Construction of Hormones

The women in the study were also asked what words came to mind when they thought about hormones and how they would draw hormones if asked to do so. The main response was for women to say that hormones "make you act crazy" or "make you too emotional." One woman said that she associated hormones with PMS (premenstrual syndrome). She said, "Hormones start rushing around in your mind, and your emotions run off course. One minute you are happy; the next you are crying. . . . And you don't even know what you are crying about." Another woman said that the word "hormones" reminded her of being sixteen years old. She said, "It makes me think of puberty with hormones raging through your body. They cause you to get your period and pimples and oily skin."

When asked how they would draw hormones, the most common response was for women to say that they would draw a human body with hormones represented by "specks" sketched across the body. One woman said that she would draw a picture of a brain "sending signals" to other parts of the body to "make hormones." Many women also said that they had heard of hormones, but they really did not know what they did or what they looked like. They saw hormones as a negative thing to be avoided.

There was some variation in the social construction of hormones by race. Euro-American or white women saw hormones as needing to be controlled. They referred to hormones "overtaking" a person's rational self and causing him or her to become irrational. Although these same women referred to menopause as natural, they still saw hormones as something to restrain. In contrast, African American or black women constructed hormones as natural parts of natural processes. For example, Yvonne said:

> Hormones are everywhere in your body. They are responsible for PMS and your emotions going haywire. Don't fight it though. You are better off if you just let menopause . . . go . . . through you as it is supposed to be. Maybe women are supposed to go through all of that and have a good cry at menopause. Women spend so much money trying to prevent menopause instead of just living through it.

The women in this study did not have extensive knowledge of hormones or what they did, despite the fact that it was the imbalance of hormones that brought on their menopausal symptoms. Knowledge of how hormones work may have been detail that was too fine to bother understanding. None of the women mentioned *male* hormones or the fact that hormones are responsible for gendered bodies and behaviors and other positive impacts in the human body.

The social construction of hormones was consistent with that of menopause. White women saw both as something to overcome, to conquer despite seeing them as a natural part of the life course. Although some women had symptoms that were so severe that they needed to be assuaged, other women attempted to constrain symptoms even before they started or when they were relatively mild. Although women constructed menopause as natural, they were not prepared to let it run its course. Many illnesses are cast in military terms. We talk about "conquering" illness and disease "invading" our bodies.[19] Menopause was not cast in such extreme terms, but white women did want to constrain the symptoms. In contrast, African American women had a more positive view of menopause and constructed hormones as a natural part of a natural process.

CONCLUSION

Race influences the experience of menopause. Many black women did not seek a doctor's assistance while undergoing menopause. Concerned that they would be given an unwelcome hysterectomy or that they would be part of a medical experiment without their permission, black women discouraged one another from going to a doctor for menopausal symptoms. Their mothers had also not gone to a doctor for menopause. Older black women hold an important role in their culture as the strong female matriarch. Menopause, as a sign of aging, then, did not imply a loss of status for them. As a result, black women reported fewer symptoms of menopause than white women. While black women mentioned hot flashes and night sweats, they did not emphasize their frequency and intensity. Instead, black women downplayed the disruption to their lives relative to other concerns. These findings are also similar to those in the literature, which suggest that black women wish to distance themselves from white women, whom they see as less resilient and less able to endure hardship.

Latina women offered two disparate social constructions of menopause. Some women saw menopause as something they should combat or conquer. They spoke glibly about not allowing it to upset their lives. They did not mention controlling their hormones, but they did see the need to steel themselves against symptoms such as hot flashes.

In contrast, a second group of Latina women avoided discussing their experience because they did not want to bring attention to their aging bodies. They thought they should allow menopause to happen as it was supposed to, without trying to control symptoms. They were particularly concerned about weight gain and losing their attractiveness, though. This may have been a reflection of the dominance of men in a machismo culture and the diminished status of postreproductive women.

The social construction of postmenopausal women as losing status needs to be changed. Women live long enough today so that half of their adult lives occur after menopause. There are many contributions that they will continue to make to the world. Most of the women in the current and future generations will have another ten years in the workforce at least. As importantly, their experience and wisdom make them optimal mentors for younger generations, and their retirement status allows them to provide many necessary services and roles that we would otherwise lose.

The medical community also needs to provide the necessary reassurance to black women so that they feel comfortable seeing a physician or other provider. Though a minority of the black women did go to a doctor when necessary, the majority did not. This leaves them vulnerable to untreated conditions that may worsen. Black women in particular have high rates of fibroids that can worsen over time, leading to complications. Many medical schools now provide sensitivity training to students who will go on to treat patients from other countries who may not speak English. That training needs to be extended to understanding black women's fears of unnecessary hysterectomies and experimentation as well as to their distinct menopausal experience.

SIX

Changing Bodies, Changing Minds

Earlier we discussed how younger women have turned to "natural" remedies for the symptoms of menopause. This includes improving nutrition, increasing exercise, and turning to Eastern traditions such as acupuncture. Young women also cite the use of phytoestrogens such as soy and bioidentical hormones to manage menopausal symptoms. Other alternatives to HRT and pharmacological treatments for menopause include the use of meditation, mindfulness, and psychotherapy to address women's needs during menopause. This chapter will focus on these latter treatments.

WOMEN'S PSYCHOSOCIAL NEEDS AT MENOPAUSE

Physician Christiane Northrup writes regarding menopause, "Our hormones are giving us the chance to see what we need to change in order to live honestly, joyfully, and fully."[1] There are a number of psychosocial needs that middle-aged women often need to address during the menopausal years. High on the list is the need to address unresolved conflict. Women often "shelve" difficult emotions and conflict during their early marital and child-rearing years when the need to focus on raising a family and building a career take precedent. Difficult emotions might include conflict with another family member, suppression of one's own needs for the good of the family, or putting professional growth on hold. Women are freer to focus on these concerns once their children have left home and their careers are further along.

Many women rethink their priorities during menopause. This could include starting a different career that would be more fulfilling but make less money, starting a long-desired hobby such as playing a musical instrument, or focusing on one's career over family needs. Having fewer responsibilities, such as raising children or paying for college tuition, makes these new priorities possible. Having seniority at work or no longer having elderly parents to care for also makes these new interests feasible. Some women may also wish to divorce during this time period, now that their children have left home, or they may wish to move to a new environment once their children are not in school. Men and women can also choose to jointly occupy roles in the home now that there is less need for a highly efficient division of labor. Postmenopausal women typically become more outspoken as a result of having fought for their needs earlier in life.

Menopausal and postmenopausal women may also aspire to change lifestyles or ways of doing things that no longer work for them. Their relationship with their spouse becomes the center of their lives now that their children are out of the home. They may desire to finally address a difficult relationship with a family member now that they no longer have to worry about the effect on their children. They might also leave an abusive or unsatisfactory marriage.

Finally, many women suffer from mood swings and depression during menopause.[2] Psychospiritual alternatives have been found to be effective in addressing these conditions as well as psychiatric disorders. Mindfulness and mediation enhance neuroplasticity, which allows the brain to change and form new ways of thinking. Advances in neuroscience have helped us to better understand why these needs arise during menopause.

USE OF MEDITATION AND MINDFULNESS FOR MENOPAUSAL SYMPTOMS

Recent findings suggest that mindfulness training and meditation are as effective as psychotherapy and antidepressants in treating psychiatric disorders. In a meta-analysis that looked at 142 randomized clinical trials involving more than 12,000 people with psychiatric disorders, Goldberg et al. found that these mindfulness-based interventions were as helpful as recognized therapies such as cognitive behavioral therapy (CBT) and pharmaceuticals.[3] The effectiveness of mindfulness for *specific* disorders was inconclusive, however. Likewise, research by the premier mindfulness advocate and trainer in the United States, Jonathan Kabat-Zinn, and others has found that mindfulness-based stress reduction (MBSR) can also cut the risk of a relapse of depression in half among those who have had three or more episodes of depression.[4] These and other findings lend credibility to the use of mindfulness-based training during menopause, when depression and mood disorders may appear.

How does mindfulness-based training effectively treat psychologically-based conditions, such as depression, or help people to deal with difficult emotions? Mindfulness is an awareness that arises through paying attention to one's thoughts on purpose, in the present, nonjudgmentally. The intention is to notice what arises in the mind while concentrating on the intake and outtake of the breath. Practitioners notice their thoughts with an open curiosity and accept them rather than dismissing them or pushing them into their subconscious. By recognizing the emotions and thoughts that they are usually too busy to discern, they are better able to work through them. Meditation also trains the practitioner to take a moment before reacting to thoughts or emotions, thus creating the space to select a healthier response than if one's mind were still on autopilot.[5,6]

According to one of the lead psychologists using mindfulness-based training, much of the pain and suffering that we experience as human beings comes from being at war with our obsessive thinking, perfectionism, attempt to control others, and retreat to false refuges such as the internet. Mindfulness teaches us to be in the present moment rather than get caught up in the stories we tell ourselves. It trains us to stop trying to be in control and instead let things be as they are. We are able to find alternative ways of understanding a problem by accepting our situation rather than resisting it.[7]

Mindfulness allows us to sit with uncomfortable thoughts rather than trying to change our condition. To that extent, it permits one to find ways to reconcile unresolved conflict, consider new options, and allow a situation to be as it is rather than trying to change it. We allow our thoughts and emotions to flow through us rather than being caught in them. This, then, decreases the likelihood of depression and ruminating.[8]

How does this happen? Research shows that meditation activates the frontal lobe of the brain. The frontal lobe is what allows you to work through emotions and to have access to your emotional landscape from which you can respond. Meditation also calms the potential for a flight or fight response in the amygdala. Meditation then makes it possible to avoid a quick reaction and to process the emotion instead.[9,10,11] See Appendix B: Meditations for Working with Difficult Emotions.

Mindfulness is also able to change our thinking through a process referred to as neuroplasticity. Rather than our brains being static organs, the structure of the brain is able to change physically over time. For example, various parts of the brain can transfer activity to a different location. The brain can also increase the amount of gray matter that it holds. Likewise, synapses between neurons can be strengthened or weakened. That is, overreactive patterns can be reversed. For example, rather than seeing an event through a negative lens, we can train our brains to impose instead a more positive lens on the experience by pausing when we notice a negative thought and instead replacing it with a more positive appraisal. We create a new neural pathway and make it the de facto thought pattern when we practice it over and over again. The more often you repeat a thought or action, the stronger the new neural pathway becomes and the more often that more positive thought or action can occur. As negative thought patterns weaken, they no longer obscure the beneficial mind states. Over time, the mind becomes accustomed to clarity, and we learn to make wiser decisions. This neuroplasticity allows us to reconsider a negative event in a new light, to review life choices without becoming bogged down in one way of thinking, and to overcome anxiety.[12,13,14,15,16]

It takes several months for the neural circuits that carry a new habit or way of thinking to consolidate fully. Practicing a new way of thinking over and over again will help ensure that you have wired it into your brain. A concentrated mind allows one to cut through a myriad of alternatives and release old patterns that cause harm to ourselves or others. Knowing that we are making a choice for our own well-being can give us the courage to take a challenging step that we might not have previously considered.[17]

Mindfulness can be used to treat other symptoms of menopause as well. In particular, mindfulness has been shown to reduce the stress associated with hot flashes and improves the physical, psychosocial, and sexual functioning of the practitioner. It improves women's resilience to the symptoms of menopause as well as the severity of some symptoms as well. While hot flash intensity did not differ significantly between women who practiced mindfulness and those who did not, the training group reported better sleep, less anxiety, and less perceived stress. In other words, it reduces the bother of menopause.[18] See Appendix D: Resources for Meditation and Mindfulness.

WHY DO THESE CHANGES OCCUR AT MENOPAUSE?

Earlier we discussed how changes in the household and work precipitate a woman's decision to rethink her priorities at midlife. How, though, does menopause specifically increase the need to address unresolved conflict or rethink priorities? Why does this process of self-reflection occur at menopause? Christiane Northrup argues that a woman's brain "catches fire" at menopause. Menopause is a reclamation process during which women get in touch with the anger that has risen from unmet and unacknowledged needs. Acknowledging and expressing that anger often leads to long overdue change. Northrup explains, "The escalation of symptoms is really our inner guidance system trying to get us to pay attention to the adjustments we need to make in our lives."[19] How though does the brain do this?

This change in the brain begins at perimenopause. Different relative levels of progesterone versus estrogen affect the temporal lobe, which is the site of enhanced intuition. Women who are experienced at mindfulness will use that enhanced intuition to recognize long-buried needs and desires and to see more clearly the changes they need to make in their lives to meet those needs. They must be willing and prepared to make those changes though, which comes from the acceptance and openness cultivated with mindfulness. Menopausal women can also use their enhanced intuition to work through unresolved conflict that comes to the surface during the practice of mindfulness.[20]

Additional changes take place at menopause. Different levels of hormones including progesterone, estrogen, FSH, and gonadotropin-releasing hormone (GnRH) affect the limbic areas, making us anxious, irritable, and emotionally volatile. The limbic system, which houses our emotional lives, supports behavior, motivation, and long-term memory along with emotions. Previously referred to as the limbic lobe, it includes the hippocampus, amygdala, thalamus and hypothalamus, and basal ganglia. During perimenopause, GnRH levels rise in the brain, causing FSH levels to surge. These drive the changes that take place in the brain. In particular, they prime the brain for new perceptions and new behaviors. We are better able to recognize our own genuine need and to understand and express anger that was not possible before. The rewiring of the female brain makes a woman's vision clearer and her motivations easier to understand. Estrogen and progesterone also bind themselves to the amygdala and hippocampus, which are responsible for memory and anger.[21] These emotions and thoughts are brought to the surface, where they can be processed. Tending to our emotions is critical because of the implications of stress and the cortisol that stress produces for the heart, cardiovascular system, and immune system. Health is enhanced when we allow our emotions to wash in and out like the tides of the sea, cleansing our minds and bodies. In contrast, feelings of powerlessness in personal relationships that get stuck and an inability to express a full range of emotions raise the risk of developing breast cancer in women and lower the survival rate from it.[22]

CASE STUDIES

Several women used mindfulness and/or psychotherapy, also referred to as talk therapy, to address unresolved conflict and to consider new priorities while going through menopause. They used these tools to address marital conflict, fears from the past, reconciling divorce, and managing depression.

Marital Conflict

Rose and her husband, Ed, raised three sons and built a family business before Rose started perimenopause. Rose said that prior to menopause, she would have said that she and Ed had a good marriage with minimal conflict. Rose left her job as a registered nurse (or RN) when Ed asked her to help him in a business that he was establishing to sell home medical equipment. Rose believed that she made that change willingly and without resentment.

Rose started having hot flashes and difficulty sleeping during perimenopause. She also remembered becoming short-tempered with Ed at that time. Rose started noticing Ed's shortcomings and questioned some of the decisions he made in their business, although she did not tell him any of this. Rose decided to see a therapist when her irritability with Ed escalated.

Rose said that she was not able to pinpoint the source of her irritability with Ed during her first sessions with her therapist. She began to notice her own resentment, though, when the therapist asked her questions about her work history and the decision to assist Ed in his business. Rose became aware that she had not wanted to leave her career as a nurse, but she did so out of a habit of always putting the needs of her husband and her children first. Likewise, Rose began to notice that Ed did not offer her any support when she was experiencing hot flashes from menopause. Rose started to understand that Ed had been taking her for granted for longer than she cared to realize.

It took Rose additional therapy to voice her concerns to Ed. Doing so allowed her to let go of her anger and to speak up for her own needs more often. Rose said:

> I don't know if I would still be married if it was not for that therapist. She helped me to see why I was so angry . . . where it came from. She started by asking me where I felt the anger in my body and what it felt like. She told me to pay attention when I started to feel it at home . . . and to ask myself what I was angry about. . . . I had been telling myself for so long that I did not mind giving up my career, but even saying it that way tells me something . . . now. Now I know how to recognize when I feel like my needs are being ignored or side-lined . . . and I can speak up for myself. . . . If it had not been for those hot flashes, I probably would have never become irritable enough to even go to a therapist. . . . Now I feel like my marriage is better, and we consider one another's opinions more.

Changing Priorities

A number of the women decided to make significant changes in their lives as a result of recognizing the desire to do so in meditation. Some of these changes were related to their work, which is discussed below. However, some were related to other facets of their lives as well. For example, Ellen decided to go from being an omnivore to a vegetarian as a result of menopause and mindfulness. She said that she started paying attention to her diet and doing research on soy and other plant-based foods to treat her hot flashes when she was perimenopausal. She started thinking about her own desire to be a vegetarian but knew that her husband would not go along with it. She said:

> I started to notice during my [meditation] practice that I was resentful of my husband . . . that his wanting to eat meat most nights shouldn't be more important than me wanting to be a vegetarian. After all, being vegetarian is healthier for you than being a red meat–eater. So I decided that my needs were important too. So now I have tried to meet him in the middle. We have more nights than we used

to when we have something vegetarian, but I make sure that it is high in protein since that is important to both of us. . . . And when I do make him a meat entrée, I make something vegetarian for myself as well. Before I would not have taken the time to do that, but I realize that I was resentful that I hadn't done that for myself. . . . Yes, I first recognized that resentment during meditation.

Similarly, Sharon recognized that she felt resentment toward people who sometimes took advantage of her during her meditation sessions around menopause. She shared with me the following:

I realized how angry I always am . . . through mindfulness. So then I went deeper to look at what was causing my anger. I realized that I often end up accommodating other people's needs rather than holding firm on my own needs. It happens a lot in the volunteer work that I do. . . . I will go along with meeting at a time that isn't good for me just to agree on a time that we *can* [Sharon's emphasis] meet. . . . I also started to notice how often I had angry thoughts when people would ask favors of me because my husband works at [a popular facility] and can get tickets for them. It is a pet peeve I have or a boundary issue, and I noticed how much it came up in my [meditation] practice.

Fear of Loss

Nina anticipated that hot flashes, vaginal dryness, and moodiness would be the first symptoms of perimenopause. Instead, her first perimenopausal symptoms were anxiety, depression, and mania. Nina was experiencing panic attacks and what she later learned was post-traumatic stress disorder (PTSD) from the earlier death of her first husband. Nina explained:

I was a different person. People told me things I said, and I couldn't believe it. I mean, I believed them, of course, but it just wasn't me. . . . I had a number of behavioral changes. I was convinced that my [second] husband was going to be killed in a car crash when he was on a trip. . . .[23] I was experiencing severe PTSD attacks. I refused to get on a plane. . . . I had to leave work for two to three weeks. I just completely shut down and was paralyzed. . . . I had to see a therapist. There were things from the past that I had to deal with . . . that I hadn't dealt with. . . . Eventually I gained control of my mental health and became myself again.

Nina would not feel herself again, though, without turning to a number of Eastern health practices. Her son suggested that she pursue mindfulness and yoga, so she found a mindfulness coach and Kundalini yoga instructor. Nina explained:

> They saved my life, the things my son suggested. It helped me to hear what my body was telling me . . . what my mind was telling me. I had never dealt with my first husband's death. . . . I was too busy making sure that my kids were okay and making ends meet. The stress at work and the hormone fluctuations brought it all to fruition. . . . My psychiatric NP suggested that I get tested for how far along I was in menopause . . . so I took a blood test. Sure enough, I was going through menopause. My body was trying to tell me that I needed to handle the rest of my life so I could handle the menopause.

Nina's son suggested that she also see a naturalist and acupuncturist. He told her that the acupuncturist could help her to get her body systems stabilized and that the naturopath could suggest natural alternatives for menopausal symptoms. The naturopath suggested taking melatonin for her insomnia and arrow root and soy for the mood swings and irritability. Nina believed that these phytoestrogens and the visits to the acupuncturist, along with the psychotherapy she received and the mindfulness and yoga practices she pursued, helped her to get her mental health under control. Nina saw her acupuncturist every other week during that time and still continues to see him once per month.

Nina also sought the support of her minister during this time. She was distressed that her husband did not understand her anxiety and mood swings. She asked her minister to speak to her husband about the need to comfort her and validate her menopausal symptoms, which her minister did during a visit to Nina's home. Nina said that it helped her significantly to have her husband's support, and she appreciated her minister's intervention.

Depression

Cynthia began noticing signs of depression in early 2014 at fifty-two years of age. She said that she felt disconnected from those around her including her husband, mother, and friends. She explained:

> I felt dead inside. I did not care about anyone or anything. I felt alone at work. I kept to myself. I did not want to socialize and avoided

having to talk to others. . . . I called my mother once a week, because I felt obligated. The rest of the time I was angry. . . . And my husband, I felt like he just wasn't interested. If I wanted to sit together on the couch, he complained that I was lying on his arm. He stayed up late watching TV while I went to bed early. I was so lonely.

It wasn't until Cynthia was stopped by a police officer on two separate occasions within one month that she realized she needed a therapist. Each occasion led to belligerent arguments with the officer. Still, she put it off, hoping that the depression would go away with the start of summer and convincing herself that the officers were in the wrong. She finally made the call to a therapist when she felt resentment at every moment of her mother and stepfather's visit during the Fourth of July weekend.

Cynthia called her insurance company to get the name of a therapist. Surprisingly, they gave her only one name and phone number, which she called.[24] She felt some relief when she had an appointment with a psychiatric nurse practitioner within a few weeks.

Cynthia's first appointment with the nurse practitioner went well. She gave her personal history and told the nurse the various SSRIs she had tried and her current dosage. It felt good to put all her problems on the table and to feel that there was someone who would help her. The nurse practitioner, Sadie, suggested that she increase the dosage of her antidepressant by only a small amount because it would be difficult to decrease the dosage later. Sadie told Cynthia that there was a good chance that she had started to go through menopause, given her age. She explained that often women have unresolved issues from earlier in life that they have not addressed. She suggested that Sadie see one of the therapists on their staff.[25]

Cynthia started seeing Julie, the therapist she was assigned to, within a few weeks. They would see one another for over one year. Cynthia said that her depression plummeted after several weeks. In fact, she felt that she was the happiest she had ever been. Julie taught Cynthia the importance of connecting with others and the need to renew her friendships. She also taught Cynthia how to reconnect with her husband through increased sex. Cynthia said that it was the first time that she saw her sex life as a positive component of her life. According to Cynthia, though, the improvement in her mood was only temporary. She was four months into her therapy when her depression returned, but this time it was worse.

Cynthia also decided to see her gynecologist to discuss the possibility of starting HRT. If her depression was due to menopause, she thought that perhaps there was some medication that she could take. Cynthia's blood work showed that she was perimenopausal, but it was not high enough to suggest that she was postmenopausal. She asked if she could try HRT to deal with her depression and (by then) hot flashes and mood swings. Cynthia's gynecologist told her that HRT would not help her because she was already well underway in the menopausal process. The doctor pointed out that what would most often be prescribed for a situation like hers was the SNRI that she was already taking, Venlafaxine™. Cynthia said that she left the doctor's office feeling disappointed.

Cynthia read every self-help book she could find, especially the ones about finding happiness. One of the books mentioned the importance of meditation as a way to increase the neuroplasticity of the mind. Cynthia said she was inspired when she read that practitioners of meditation can retrain their brains to have more positive thoughts than negative ones by strengthening the neural pathways of positive thoughts. Cynthia thought that this sounded perfect for her and looked on the internet for meditation classes in her geographical area. She soon learned that there were classes for meditation-based stress reduction at the nearby university. Cynthia immediately signed up for their eight-week course.

Cynthia said that mindfulness training changed her life. Becoming more mindful of her thoughts helped her to see that her problems with her mother had not been resolved in her therapy with Julie. She found a second therapist who helped her to realize that she suffered from maternal attachment disorder, a condition that had caused great unhappiness and a feeling of loss for many years. Between the mindfulness training and her therapy, Cynthia was able to accept her relationship with her mother for what it was and to recognize that she no longer needed a mother or mother replacement. Cynthia said that it was not until four or five years after her first appointment with the nurse practitioner, Sadie, that she believed that her depression was well behind her. Cynthia said that her nurse practitioner had been right all along and that her unresolved issue with her mother had surfaced with the hormonal fluctuations of perimenopause. Her mood swings brought her to therapy and then the combination of therapy and mindfulness. It was the interaction of these two things that allowed Cynthia to understand her disorder and to prevent it from continuing to debilitate her. She added:

Mindfulness changed my life. I don't know where I would be today if I had not stumbled upon it. I can see now that the depression I have had for a long time was due to my problems with my mother. I have even been able to wean myself off my antidepressants by knowing why I get depressed and learning to interact with my mother in a healthier way rather than just increasing my medication every six months. . . . Taking that class, doing all the reading, and continuing the practice made all the difference. . . . I wouldn't have stumbled upon it if I had not gone to therapy, and I would not have gone to therapy if I wasn't going through menopause.

THE IMPACT OF MENOPAUSE OVERALL ON WORK

Menopause affected women's work in a myriad of ways. Many of the women said that no longer menstruating had a very positive effect on their work life. For example, Susan said that no longer getting PMS (premenstrual syndrome) had a very positive impact on her career. Susan had drifted from one job to another throughout her adulthood. She said that she had a very difficult time getting along with her coworkers and that she would periodically "blow up" at them. It was only when she had completed menopause that she realized her outbursts were probably linked to PMS. She explained:

> I am not sure if I ever recognized that my blow-ups were because of PMS . . . or that I knew several days later [after the incident], but I just could not control my temper when it happened. Either way, I have been bouncing through jobs my whole life because I made enemies. That has not happened since menopause, though. I am much, much calmer and don't have the highs and lows that I used to get. . . . I can finally stay at one job and start to get seniority and make some friends.

Likewise, Priscilla said that she had missed a significant amount of work over the years because of heavy periods. Being postmenopausal meant that she no longer had to worry about missing so much work. She said, "I used to have such bad periods in my thirties that I would vomit. I was always worried that I was going to start throwing up and felt like I had to leave work as soon as I started feeling queasy. Plus, I was always bloated and just wanted to get home through my whole period. I didn't want to be at work." Later she also added:

> When I had my periods, I could never go on overnight trips for work. My periods were just so bad that I did not want to be away from work

when they came. . . . I worried that my boss thought I just didn't want to take advantage of opportunities to advance. . . . But what would I do if I was at some meeting in another city with my colleagues and couldn't control the bleeding. I don't even stay at bed-and-breakfast places on vacation because I am worried that I will bleed on the sheets and bedding.

Beth said that she was always tired when she had her periods. Other women said that they sometimes felt that they had "brain fog." Kelsey added, "I used to have such a hard time speaking in front of people at work when I had my periods because I would get tongue-tied. I couldn't think of the right word, and I would feel like an idiot." The vast majority of the women said that they had much more energy in their postmenopause years that they could devote to work. Cynthia said:

I wake up, and I can't wait to get to work. . . . I used to be a sluggard, just dragging myself through the day. Since menopause, I am just fly-ing though. I don't mind bringing work home with me. I have the energy to do it whereas I didn't in the past. . . . I am really enjoying work so much more than I ever did. I feel like I am really at my peak now . . . like I am fully alive.

Joy pointed out that she has much more confidence since going through menopause. She believed that this confidence carried over into the work-place as well. She explained:

Making it through menopause . . . realizing that you are in with the senior people at work . . . it gives you more confidence. I know that no matter what comes up at work, I can figure out how to deal with it or fix it. . . . I got through menopause . . . I can get through anything.

Mindfulness and Work

Women who practiced meditation and mindfulness found it useful in resolving conflict at work and considering changes to their careers. Vicki was an experienced practitioner of meditation and mindfulness before she entered perimenopause. It was not until perimenopause though that she began to notice that she was unhappy. As she approached those thoughts with an open curiosity, she began to also notice that she was questioning her role in her current job and whether or not she was able to be effective at it. She noticed more thoughts about seeking alternative jobs, and she even noted that she was rehearsing how she might tell her current boss that she intended to leave. Vicki said:

> I started having brainstorms about new jobs that I could do with the work skills that I had and how much happier I would be. I never considered these other jobs or how I could apply what I do now to those [jobs], but all of a sudden it came to me . . . I know mindfulness is supposed to help you to do that . . . to find the solutions when you are able to clear your mind and stuff . . . and it worked. . . . I think also because of menopause, I was asking myself, "Is this the kind of career that I want to have for myself for the rest of my life?" It was on the tip of my mind . . . but I had never really realized how unhappy I was in my job before this.

Ellen said that the practice of meditation around menopause helped her to decide to go back to school in preparation for a new career. She explained:

> I got really interested in nutrition, using herbs, plant-based diet and that kind of thing while I was going through menopause. I was doing it for my own needs, but I realized how much I liked it. . . . It was during meditation when I realized just how much I liked thinking about good nutrition and how much I wanted to go back to school. . . . So that is what I am doing now, going back to school and studying to be a nutritionist.

Kathy decided during menopause that she wanted to change from full-time to part-time work so that she could do more of the things that she enjoyed. She said, "Menopause made me realize that I am middle-aged now and that maybe it is time for a change. I feel like I have earned the right to take some time off to spend with my grandchildren. . . . I meditated on it and made the decision."

Similarly, Karen was still premenopausal but had decided to quit her job completely in order to concentrate on other things in her life. Karen said that it was while she was meditating that she realized that although she was not unhappy, she wanted to do something else with her work. She said:

> I kept having thoughts of other things I wished I was doing with my time rather than going to work every day. I really get a great deal of satisfaction from the community service that I do, but my paid work was making it difficult for me to invest further of myself into that. So I waited for about six months after I was noticing those thoughts, and then I handed in my early retirement . . . letter.

CONCLUSION

Christiane Northrup, MD, argues that menopause sets the female brain on fire. She states, "Our hormones are giving us the chance to see what we need to change in order to live honestly, fully, joyfully, and healthfully in the second half of our lives."[26] The changing relative levels of progesterone versus estrogen affect (1) the temporal lobe of the brain, resulting in an enhanced intuition, and (2) the limbic system, which regulates our emotions and behaviors. Menopausal women are thus better able to see the causes of unresolved conflict from the past and respond to those causes positively. They are able to see how they might wish to reprioritize the second half of their adult lives in order to live more fully and authentically. They are able to recognize their emotions and make the changes in their lives that they were not able to do when they were younger and focused on their children and building a career.

Many women effectively use mindfulness and meditation practice as well as psychotherapy to assist them in this process. Mindfulness is the awareness that arises when we pay attention deliberately to our thoughts with open curiosity and acceptance in the present. This open curiosity and acceptance allows women to work more effectively with painful areas of their lives or unpleasant thoughts to make needed changes. Therapy, in many ways, does the same thing, with the therapist providing support while helping patients to see more clearly the causes of their pain. Menopause thus creates the changes to the brain that allow women to use mindfulness practice and psychotherapy to treat some of the symptoms of menopause or to at least manage them while also allowing women to make necessary changes in their lives in order to live fully.

SEVEN

Marriage, Sex, and Family Relationships

MARRIAGE

Menopause can be a difficult time for marriages. Wives must learn to deal with hot flashes and night sweats while their emotions and hormones are rapidly fluctuating. They may feel less attractive as their bodies and weight change. Some may wonder what impact this will have on their marriages. Husbands—or wives—may feel like they are walking on egg shells. In an ideal situation, the other spouse will try to minimize stressors from children and elderly parents, but not all spouses may be aware of the need or advantage of doing so.

While menopause does affect marriage, it is important to note that marriage also alters menopause. First, let us look at the impact of menopause on marriage. In a survey of 326 midlife women, researchers found a significant negative correlation between marital satisfaction and menopause symptoms. As menopausal symptoms went up, marital satisfaction went down. When symptoms such as hot flashes and night sweats increased, anger and depression increased as well, making it more difficult to maintain a happy marriage. However, married women reported fewer feelings of depression, suggesting that marriage can also guard against some menopausal symptoms. Marriage can offer resilience against the challenges of life, including menopause.[1]

The quality of the marriage, though, is an important factor. A supportive, low-stress marriage reduced the strain of menopause and made the symptoms less severe and easier to manage. However, women in dissatisfying marriages, characterized by less social support, less depth, and higher conflict, reported increased stress and more symptoms than women in satisfying marriages.[2]

MENOPAUSE AND WELL-BEING

Rates of depression among women are relatively high in midlife. High levels of menopausal symptoms can lead to decreased mental wellbeing and lower perceived quality of life.[3] Yet, menopause is not the only thing causing depression among women. Caring for elderly parents and minor children, whether separately or simultaneously, and work-related stress can also cause depression among women. However, menopause is often the assumed culprit of these issues rather than the other challenges at this time of life. As mentioned above, satisfying marriages can be a buffer for the effect of menopause on well-being. If it is a thriving marriage in which the wife feels supported, menopause will not necessarily reduce well-being. For this reason, it is important for husbands to continue to be supportive of their wives during menopause.

The relationship between menopausal symptoms and stress is bidirectional. Just as menopausal symptoms can increase stress at midlife, life stresses can also worsen menopausal symptoms. For example, a less satisfying marriage, which can be stressful, is related to greater menopausal symptomology.[4] For this reason, it is even more important that women use the enhanced intuition and greater focus on their personal lives that come in perimenopause to address unresolved issues in their marriage and strengthen their primary bond. As was argued earlier in this book, mindfulness training and sometimes even psychotherapy can optimize the likelihood of this occurring.

FINDINGS

Menopause and Marriage

Results of this study show that menopause does affect marriage. In fact, there are multiple avenues for direct and indirect effects of menopause on marital quality and the likelihood of divorce. Several of the women said that their husbands were not particularly supportive of them as they went through menopause and that the men "blamed" the things that their wives did on being menopausal. For example, Susan and her husband were retired. Every time that Susan became emotional or changed her mind about something, her husband, Chuck, would say that it was due to menopause. According to Susan, though, her menopausal symptoms had been over for years. Yet, Chuck chose to see her behavior as a symptom of menopause. Likewise, Karen's husband was angry that Karen had become more vocal about her thoughts during perimenopause and that she was more likely to express her opinion. He said that menopause had made her into one of those "women's libbers."

The impact on the women's marriages had more to do with how they responded to their husband's reactions than to the husband's reactions themselves. Susan, for example, found Chuck's comments that she was emotional and changing her mind because of menopause as humorous. She laughed at the fact that either he was unaware that she was no longer going through menopause or that he was unaware that she had always been emotional and likely to change her mind. In fact, she found this lack of awareness to be an endearing quality in her husband. She said, "Honestly, you gotta love the big lug head." In contrast, Karen was furious that her husband took issue with her increased assertiveness, which she saw as a positive change. She said, "I couldn't believe that he would be *threatened* [her emphasis] by my sticking up for myself every now and then . . . rather than being a doormat. He made *all* the decisions, and I was just trying to get him to consider my thoughts."

Karen did eventually divorce her husband after menopause. She said that menopause itself did not cause the divorce, but that her husband's lack of support for her during menopause and his reaction to her new self-assertion did play a part in it. She said, "The real cause of the divorce was that the kids were gone, and we realized just how much we had drifted apart. . . . He hadn't been there for me when my dad was dying and my mother needed me more than he did. . . . It made menopause so much harder than it had to be."

Martha and her husband, Ron, also divorced after menopause. Martha said that she decided during perimenopause that she wanted to lose all the weight that she gained after her children were born. Martha became more aware of just how much this weight gain had plagued her and prevented her from becoming the person she wished to be. She became much more self-confident and outgoing as a result of the weight loss, though. She explained:

I realized that my husband was a good friend, but I was no longer *in love* [her emphasis] with him. He was my first love . . . but I wanted more now. I wanted someone who cared how he looked for his wife, who was willing to work out. My husband was a couch potato. . . . I guess you could say we had gone our separate ways.

The effects of menopause on marriage were not all negative, though. Several of the women said that their marriages were actually stronger after menopause because they appreciated their husband's support throughout the process. Rose said:

> That poor guy. He went through hell with my menopause. First the heat was up, and then it was down. Then I was opening all of the windows in the dead of winter. . . . At night I tossed and turned . . . and I tossed and turned. I would kick the covers so far off that I kicked them off his side, too. . . . He would just say, "It's going to be okay. Don't worry about it." But I felt bad. . . . Plus, my emotions were all over the place. I would cry at the drop of a hat. . . . He would just hug me, though, and say it was okay.

Kathy also appreciated how supportive her husband was during menopause. She explained:

> I am surprised the neighbors never called the police with all the yelling I did. It was that bad. Steve just took it in stride, though. He would tell the kids, "Your mom is having a bad day. Just leave her alone, and she will be fine. . . . Just don't say anything though. . . ." Then he and I would go out . . . get out of the house . . . and usually I would feel better.

She added later in the interview:

> It is one of those things that either pulls you together and makes you stronger, or it tears you apart. For us, it made us closer. We can laugh about it now. . . . But seriously, I now know that I can depend on Steve no matter what. Not that I didn't know that before, but it just . . . confirmed it for me.

Other women said that menopause "forced" them to work out the problems in their marriages. For example, Cynthia started practicing mindfulness and attending therapy in response to the depression that came with perimenopause. She explained:

> My therapist pointed out that I was depressed because my marriage was weak. My husband and I . . . well, our sex life had died on the

vine, so to speak. We had to get our sex life back on track, and that wasn't as easy as it seems. I had to be patient. It wasn't something that was going to happen overnight. . . . Men go through menopause, too, male menopause . . . and they have less testosterone. So they might need something like Viagra™. It is almost like you need to learn to have sex again. Neither one of us was young again. I had vaginal dryness. He had ED [erectile dysfunction]. We had both gained weight. . . . More importantly, I needed mindfulness to be aware of how to keep the love alive, how to keep the feeling of being in love alive. And how to show appreciation and willingness to put the other person first . . . and then they will put you first, too, and you get your needs met that way. It took my mindfulness practice to be self-aware enough to do all of that and not just react or be on autopilot all the time. It is about learning to be more appreciative of one another and cultivate gratitude. . . . It turned my life around. I don't know where I would be if it had not been for the mindfulness . . . and therapy.

Menopause and Well-Being

Most of the women who were postmenopausal at the time of the study believed that they possessed greater well-being after menopause than prior to perimenopause. Even the women who were divorced stated that they were in a better frame of mind than they had been before menopause. As one woman said, "Yes, I still have a few hot flashes, but it is so much better to be through that than being at the beginning and having to go through it." This is not to say that other things had not happened in their lives that saddened them,[5] but the majority believed that it was better to be postmenopausal than to be menstruating still or going through perimenopause or menopause.

Most of the postmenopausal women were still working outside of the home at the time of the study. A few had changed jobs after great deliberation during menopause. Women said that they were content and satisfied with the work that they were doing at this stage in their life. For example, Kathy said:

I am happy with what I am doing now, very happy. I used to work for a university, but they would not give me the resources that I needed to get the job done. Now I work for myself. I don't take on more [clients] than I can handle, and I get to set my own hours and my own pay. . . . I wouldn't have dared to go off on my own before, but at this stage of my life, I can afford to do so.

Kathy also took great delight in being able to spend part of her day baby-sitting for her two grandchildren when her daughter was not able to pick them up from school. She explained:

I get home early enough now that I can drive over to the kids' schools if my daughter gets stuck in traffic or has to work late. This is a great time in my life to . . . to be able to spend that time with them. We make cookies and do crafts . . . and it is just fabulous.

Other women also felt a great sense of well-being. One of the women explained:

I feel a new sense of calm . . . since menopause. I am not running around like a chicken with its head cut off. I don't know if it is because my hormones have settled down, and I am not reacting to PMS every month like I used to. I was like a bomb that would go off every month with no notice. I would be moody and irritable for days . . . then have cramps and bleeding for ten days. Now though, I don't have to worry about losing my cool, about feeling irritable or crampy. It is like you come out on the other side of menopause and life is so, so much better.

Those women who took exception to this were the ones who were upset that they could no longer conceive children and, according to them, were not as physically attractive as they had been. These women were less likely to have finished college and were part of a culture that emphasized women's value as being based on their attractiveness. Their husbands were often the primary breadwinners while the wives worked part time.

Older women, however, like older men, have important contributions to make to society. The seven women who were retired all volunteered, assisted their families, or mentored young people. One of the women was a religious education teacher for the children in one grade level at her church. She said, "It is only one hour a week with the kids, plus the time that I spend preparing, but it makes me feel good to do it. I feel like I am giving back, or maybe it is paying it forward to a new generation."

Other women also spent time with their grandchildren, teaching them how to bake from family recipes or sharing stories about family traditions.

This concern for later generations is referred to as generativity and is one of the ways older people make valuable contributions to society.[6]

Retired postmenopausal women also volunteered. One of the women was a docent or guide in an art museum. She enjoyed being able to share her passion for art with others. Other women volunteered at a food pantry, assisted in their local polling quarters, and served on the campaigns of their favorite politicians. These women made important contributions to society that younger men and women who are working outside of the home or caring for young children cannot make. While the sentiment in male-dominated societies may be that postmenopausal women lose their status with their fertility, gerontologists and those who study changes across the life course argue that older people of both genders make important contributions to society. They are better able to weigh multiple sides of an issue and thus make superior arbiters. Their enhanced wisdom and skill come from years of lived experience. They are freed from keeping pace with "the Joneses" and can focus on what is important. Older men and women are more likely to live in the present and make the most of their time on Earth.[7] Postmenopausal women should continue to enjoy the high status that is afforded of all individuals throughout life.

SEX

There is a myth in the United States that menopausal women's libido drops irrevocably because of the decrease in estrogen. According to Northrup, "This change in sex drive has absolutely nothing to do with hormone levels and everything to do with a woman's deepest unfilled desires, desires that are now rising into her consciousness."[8] Northrup points out that many women do in fact experience a decrease in their sex drive during perimenopause, but she argues that this is the result of changes in the brain that put our relationships and emotions under a microscope, including our sexual relationships. She explains, "If a woman's sexual relationship needs to be updated, if she is not getting the tenderness and care she desires, or if she has unfinished business with her mate, then any or all of these issues may well arise at this time."[9] If a woman recognizes the need to make improvements in her marriage or to update her sex life in keeping with her desires and needs, she may be able not only to get her libido back on track but to improve her marriage overall.

In contrast, other researchers have found that women experience greater enjoyment of sexual activity upon menopause. Dillaway's study of forty-five middle-class, heterosexual, menopausal women found increased enjoyment of sex in perimenopause in comparison to premenopause.[10] This may, in part, be a cohort effect or an attribute of this generation of menopausal women in particular. Another study shows that middle-aged women fifty-five and older enjoy sex more and put more thought and energy into their sex lives than women of the same age a decade ago. They are also more open about their sexual needs and consider a healthy sex life to be a part of a healthy lifestyle.[11] Another study found that midlife men and women have sex as often as younger adults (an average of two to three times a month) and that 25 percent of the oldest group (seventy-five to eighty-five years of age) are still having sex. The effect is contingent on the woman's health status, though. Women in poor health reported having sex the least.[12] Research on healthy, nonsmoking menopausal women with partners found that there is no change in sexual satisfaction, frequency of sexual intercourse, or difficulty reaching orgasm compared to premenopause.[13]

Northrup argues that a woman's thoughts and emotions have more to do with her ability to perform sexually than anything else.[14] If a woman has been able to right her marriage and feels that she has a loving and responsive sexual partner, she will be able to perform as she always has. Unresolved conflict in her marriage though will continue to fuel the dip in libido. Because of the complexity of female sexuality, drugs such as flibanserin have not been found to offer any benefit.[15] What will solve any interruption in women's sexuality, then, is the use of mindfulness and therapy to identify any unresolved issues or new needs in their sexuality. In addition, the cultural programming that depicts postmenopausal women as less desirable and of little worth also undermines their ability to enjoy their sexuality. Such toxic definitions of femininity need to be redressed in the world at large. Northrup writes, "Resolving problems in an existing relationship can have an effect on your sex life that's comparable to that of a new sex partner. . . . Hanging on to old anger and resentment, on the other hand, quells libido rapidly."[16] Thus, a woman's physical and mental health are more important to her sexual functioning than her menopausal status.

Having a healthy sex life will improve a couple's marital satisfaction overall. The hormone oxytocin, which is released by the pituitary gland during labor and breastfeeding, is released during orgasm for both men and women. Referred to as "the love hormone," oxytocin plays a significant role in bonding.

FINDINGS

Menopause and Sex

The results of this research suggest that a woman's libido may decrease during perimenopause but that it is rare for it to be irreversible. One woman believed that her libido was permanently lessened because intercourse had become painful due to vaginal dryness. However, she had tried only one treatment option for vaginal dryness at the time of the study. Other women who had vaginal dryness said that their gynecologists had prescribed an ointment to produce a natural lubrication or that they had added a lubricant during intercourse. Another woman said that she and her husband had prolonged foreplay to increase the likelihood of vaginal lubrication. In other words, most couples found a way around the side effect in order to maintain their sex life.

Other women said that they also experienced some decrease in their sex lives when they were having severe hot flashes and other menopausal symptoms. Sallie said, "The last thing you want to do is get romantic when you're having hot flashes and you can't stand to even have a cotton tee on you, never mind another hot, sweaty body." Likewise, Joy said, "I was going crazy with hot flashes. I was constantly feeling like I was at the end of my rope. Sex just wasn't on the table. Eventually, though, once I got HRT and got my hot flashes under control, we could go back to our regular sex life."

Still others said that menopause actually increased their libido. Cynthia said that she became more interested in sex after going off birth control. She explained:

At first I thought that I was losing my mind. All of a sudden I thought about sex like I did when I was a young woman. I couldn't figure it out, and then I remembered how there were always warnings on the packages of my birth control pills with statements that the pills could decrease sex drive. . . . And my gyn used to ask me about it every year, too, but I was just too self-conscious to tell him that yes, the pills had lowered my sex drive. Now I feel stupid that I, *we* [her italics] were missing out on a better sex life all of those years.

A few of the postmenopausal women said that their sex life had improved because they were just happier in general. They believed that they had fewer things to worry about and distract them compared to when they were younger. Priscilla said, "I just know myself better and know my husband better. There is more trust." Lauren said, "I don't have to worry about the kids hearing anymore. We can be more passionate. We can have sex any time of the day now. It was harder when the kids were still living at home. . . . We even had sex in the shower one day. That would not have happened in the past."

Those women who said that their marriages had improved during menopause believed that their sex lives had improved as a result. Cynthia said:

> It is night and day. My husband and I had lost our sex life. There is no other way to put it. We just got derailed. Now though . . . we are making up for lost time. Before I thought that sex came from the love, and if you lost the love, you lost the sex too. But it is actually more of a cycle. The sex makes the couple, too. It pulls you together more. . . . I realized how happy it made my husband. No one else can have that impact on his life the way I can. It is a privilege to be the one who can make him happy like that.

RELATIONSHIPS WITH EXTENDED FAMILY

Women believed that meditation and mindfulness improved their relationship with some extended family members as well. Amy said that her relationships with her adult daughter and son were much improved since she began meditation. She shared the following:

> I started meditating about ten years ago. It has made a huge difference in my relationship with my kids. My daughter used to always get mad at me. She would be telling me something on the phone about some problem she was having, and I would tell her about what I thought she should do or what I just thought, and she would get so mad at me. It happened all the time. . . . I thought it was just the way that it was . . . the way that it was always going to be. I didn't think there was any way that I could keep her from getting mad at me. . . . And then I started meditating. I realized that I thought I was *right* [Amy's emphasis], that I was always right. . . . Plus, I wasn't saying it [my advice] in a way that she could hear it. So I started being much more thoughtful . . . mindful . . . of *how* [Amy's emphasis] I was

saying things to her. I try to offer my advice as something that she might want to think about rather than telling her what is the right way to think. . . . My son . . . well, he can just be such a difficult person, and I have had to learn to just accept that. That is one of the things that they teach you in meditation . . . in Buddhism really . . . that we need to accept things as they are in the present moment rather than resisting them because that only makes the emotion stronger . . . when you try to stuff it down rather than accept it. . . . So I have had to learn to accept the things that he says rather than getting hurt. . . . I have had to accept the fact that my son and daughter don't get along, and that is just the way it is. It doesn't make me a bad mother; it is just the way it is. . . . I allow the emotion to just be. So things are better. My family is more at peace because of this mindfulness training.

Lauren was always furious at her brother because he did not want to be as close as she did. In her meditation practice, she started to recognize her anger more as hurt than as anger. She said that she started crying while she was meditating because she was thinking about how her brother did not want her to visit. Lauren realized at that point that what underlay her anger was a Band-Aid for the hurt. Lauren then started seeing a therapist who could help her to process her feelings.

Claire worked through her anger at her mother as a result of meditation. She shared with me the following:

My brother could never do anything wrong. My mother would always take his side. I would be the one to get into trouble when he did something wrong because I was older. . . . Then later she would take money that I gave her for rent and give it to my brother because he was always in some kind of trouble . . . pregnant girlfriends, gambling debts. . . . But she always defended him. Anyway, I realized that I have knocked myself out my whole life trying to get her to love me the way that she loved him. I realized that I have been trying to get her to feel the same way about me . . . love me the same way. I was always trying to please her, to do right by her. I have learned to let it go, though. . . . What a difference that has made in my life. I have felt free . . . free from knocking my head against the wall trying to get her be something she isn't. . . . Yes, I started noticing how angry I was during perimenopause, and I started seeing a therapist. My therapist has helped me to work through my feelings. She was the one who got me started on the meditation too so that I could work on . . . on myself.

Zoe: The Midlife Brain on Fire

Zoe was a professional woman who had been married for twenty-five years. Her two children had recently left home at the time of the study. Zoe believed that she was mostly happily married, but she said that had not always been the case. Zoe explained:

> It was around the time that I noticed my periods becoming very irregular. I was telling my friend that I was getting really tired of bleeding all the time, of always having to worry about tampons overflowing. She said, "It sounds like you have started menopause." She was fifty and had already been through it. . . . At one point my friend said, "I realized when I turned 50 that this is it. It isn't going to get better than this. *This* is what we have been working toward all these years—getting the kids through college, paying off the house, having two careers. . . . We need to enjoy this now. In ten years we might have health problems or sick parents. Things might get worse, but they probably won't get better than this."

Zoe said that she realized that this was true and that she needed to enjoy this period of her life, to stop and enjoy this time that she had. She said:

> I could see that I am always living a month ahead of time instead of enjoying the here and now. I could also see that I needed to put more emphasis [on] my marriage if I was going to do this. . . . My husband and I, we did not not fight, we had a good life. But we were living separate lives, and that was partially my fault. I had let it happen because I was so geared to the kids, my career, the house and laundry. Everything else had to be on autopilot.

Zoe said later in the interview that after that realization, she was reading an article that felt like it had "been written for" her. Zoe explained:

> The article said that often people are unhappy because they want to be somewhere else or someone else. It said that true happiness comes when we can be content with who we are, with where we are. . . . So I started paying attention to what relationships I had, to what I had with my husband to begin with . . . to what brought us together.

Zoe described this process of reinvigorating her marriage thus:

> It was a long process . . . we are still working on it. It is appreciating one another and not taking one another for granted. For example, I am more likely to go to a ball game with my husband than I used to because I know he enjoys it. Before, I would have gone shopping with my daughter. And he is more likely to go out for a nice dinner, just the two of us, and really listen to what I am saying. . . . I am embarrassed to say it, but my husband was depressed for a while, and I did not even know it. . . . Now I am paying attention and working to make our time together fulfilling for both of us.

CONCLUSION

Women say that menopause does impact their marriages and sex lives, but it isn't always for the worse. A few of the women left their spouses between menopause and the time of this study, or they experienced difficulty with intimacy for a while due to vaginal dryness. The majority, however, said that their marriages and sex lives were the same or better since menopause. Many said that the menopausal time period actually strengthened their marriages. They appreciated that their spouses were supportive while they went through menopause and believed that the experience had brought them closer together. Others said that they were just happier in general as both the years of menstruating and perimenopause and menopause were behind them. Many of the women also noted the need to focus more on their marriages when they saw their personal lives and relationships under a microscope during perimenopause. These women could more clearly see the need to focus on their marriages, resolve conflict, and prepare for the second half of their marriages, which would no longer include their children and their careers being the focus of attention. These women tried to recapture what had drawn them to their spouses to begin with or to build a new marriage that took into account all that they had learned about each other over the years and all the wisdom that had come with their maturity.

The majority of the women said that their sex lives improved once they passed menopause. Some of the women attributed this to the fact that they were no longer on birth control pills that had dampened their libido. Many forms of birth control include warnings of the side effects on sexual desire. Others said that having their children out of the home allowed them to focus on one another again, including their sex lives. They noted that they had the house to themselves now and could have sex where and when they wanted and no longer had to keep their passion quiet because of the children. Couples also had more time together than they had in the past.

A few of the women did feel that their sex lives suffered from menopause. One woman had not been able to effectively treat the vaginal dryness that made intercourse painful. Others felt despair that they were no longer sexually attractive and able to have children. The despair these women experienced comes from our cultural programming that defines a woman's worth according to her sexual appeal or ability to reproduce. These women tended to come from family cultures where the husband dominated. They felt that their worth was diminished as they saw little value in the other roles that older women hold in our society.

This underscores the need to change cultural programming and our preoccupation with how women look. We as a society are well past a time in which women should be defined solely by their sexual appeal and ability to reproduce. Women's postmenopausal years now claim a much larger percentage of their lives and a longer number of years than ever before. As such, they can have second careers that are not constrained by the same requirements of a first career, including the need to make enough money to raise children and buy a house. They can use the wisdom they have accrued through the years to make important contributions through civic engagement, the arts, and services that are optimally provided by women. The ability to nurture is not a deficit of womanhood but an asset that does not wane because of menopause. There are many contributions that women make in their postmenopausal years on which our society depends. We need to change our ideas of what makes women valuable beyond their attractiveness, sex appeal, and ability to reproduce to include these other contributions and attributes as well.

EIGHT

Going Deeper: Meditation to Manage Feeling Out of Control

Meditation creates changes in the brain that make it easier to work with difficult emotions that crop up in menopause or any point in life. Meditation causes the amygdala, the site of the fight-or-flight response, to calm down. It also brings online the frontal lobe, which allows the practitioner to work through emotions and access their emotional landscape. Rather than reacting to a stimulus without a chance to process it, meditation opens up a pause that allows one to respond rather than react. We become more aware of our thoughts and emotions and can trace their origins. We can recognize compulsive thinking and the negative parts of our personality that we project onto others.[1]

By calming the amygdala, meditation opens up a window that permits the practitioner to respond rather than react to anger or a trigger. However, it takes significant practice for that pause to arise. Once it does, it is such a subtle change in one's response that the meditator may not even be aware of the change. With time, though, one will notice that one is no longer reacting in anger or flying off the handle. This is particularly important for women who are feeling angry in menopause or for those who have been abused themselves and wish to break the cycle of abuse.

Creating a pause can be achieved by nearly any meditation practice. The simplest would be to anchor your attention to your breath. Sit in a relaxed, upright position. Feel yourself in your body. Imagine a rod going from the top of your head down to your "sit bones." Your hands may be relaxed at your side or lying, palms open, on your knees. Your eyes may be closed, or your gaze may be soft and cast slightly down. Begin to watch the rise and fall of your breath. Feel yourself breathing and be with your breath. Anchor your attention to your breath. As your mind starts to wander, or your attention drifts away from your breath, simply notice your thoughts as they arise and allow them to float by. Bring your attention back to your breath when it wanders away like that. It does not matter how long you have drifted off. Bring an open and accepting curiosity to your thoughts and then allow them to flow by. Together, awareness of body, breath, and mind create your meditation practice.[2]

Meditation also allows the practitioner to become more aware of the destructive triggers that send us running to false refuges such as the internet, television, shopping, eating, and consumption of alcohol and drugs. It may be toxic thoughts of not being good enough or worthy of love, or it may be emotions such as fear, envy, grief, and guilt. By noticing the thoughts that sweep through our minds, we begin to understand the underlying emotions. This gives us a place where we can start the beginning of our own self-exploration. Notable Buddhist nun Pema Chödrön argues that we constantly shield ourselves from the painful parts of our lives because they scare us. We put up protective walls of opinions, prejudices, and other barriers out of a deep fear of being hurt.[3] One of the women in the study had always stayed out of the limelight out of a deep fear that she was not as smart as the other people with whom she worked. She did not volunteer for greater responsibility at work because she was afraid that others would realize that she was not as bright as they were. This feeling of being less worthy created great suffering for the woman though.

One of the fundamental underpinnings of Buddhism is that there is always suffering. This is the first of the Four Noble Truths of Buddhism. We have to look deeply into our own suffering and see how it came to be. This arising of suffering is the Second Noble Truth. The Third Noble Truth is that healing is possible. Several Buddhists have written that in order to heal, we must recognize and be with the source of our suffering. Rather than trying to push away or attempting to escape the thing that causes us pain, such as the loss of a loved one, we must be willing to be present with it and feel it. Too often, though, we try to escape pain. We seek refuge in places and practices that do nothing to diminish the pain and may even create greater pain or shame, such as overeating, drinking or using drugs, or overspending on material goods that we do not need. It may take repeated experiences of being with our suffering or the emotions that are causing us pain before we are able to let these painful experiences and emotions go. The Fourth Noble Truth is the path that keeps us from doing the things that cause suffering. The Buddha referred to this as the Noble Eightfold Path, translated as the Path of Eight Right Practices. These practices include Right View, Right Thinking, Right Speech, Right Action, Right Livelihood, Right Diligence, Right Mindfulness, and Right Concentration. For example, by having an occupation that makes the world a better place, that does not cause harm, and that alleviates the suffering of others, we ourselves will be less likely to suffer. By using speech that is kind and compassionate and acting in ways that protect our earth and do not cause harm or suffering to others, we ourselves will be less likely to suffer. This tendency to reap what we have sown is referred to as karma.[4]

Tara Brach has adapted a meditation for managing destructive thoughts and difficult emotions for Western practitioners to use. It is referred to as the R.A.I.N. meditation. During the process of meditating, practitioners are guided (or can guide themselves) through the following four steps:

Recognize the emotion: Ask yourself, what is this thing that is making you feel badly about yourself or that is making you feel empty? Recognize the emotion and name it.

Allow (or Accept) the emotion: Allow your feelings to be just as they are. Experience the swelling of deep grief or deep pain and whisper, "I consent." Just by whispering a phrase like this, you loosen the resistance and allow yourself to be one with the emotion.

Investigate the emotion: Where do you feel this emotion? What does it feel like? What is this emotion telling you? What do you need to heal?

Nurture (or Nonidentification): Recognize that your sense of who you are is not fused with or defined by any limited set of emotions, sensations, or stories. Ask yourself how you would feel if you were not at war with yourself. Be kind to yourself and acknowledge your own innate goodness.[5]

Meditation teaches the practitioner to live in the present. The only thing that matters is what is happening right here, right now. We cannot go back and change the past, and neither can we be assured of the future. We observe each thought that is produced as a manifestation of our mind and allow it to go. In addition, the practitioner is taught not to grasp or cling to how we would like things to be but to accept them as they are. Rarely are we ever able to craft a situation to be how we would like it to be. Even if we could, there is always change, which causes external conditions to alter. The only thing that we have any control over is our own inner self. To prevent our own suffering, we must learn to live with things as they are. This helps practitioners to live more comfortably with change and uncertainty, including the ups and downs of menopause. It can be argued that this practice is what allows women to manage their hot flashes and menopause overall.[6]

Meditation can also free individuals from compulsive thinking. Buddhist psychology reminds us that our minds are always producing thoughts. It is what minds do. However, there may not be any truth to what we think. We assume that we know other people's motivations and thoughts, but Buddhism argues that there is no knowing. Our assumptions are projections of our own ego and are not based on anything concrete. Our minds create stories that we tell ourselves over and over again. These stories often free us from the responsibility of wrongdoing or make us feel superior over another person. We believe that we are the ones who know the right way of being or doing things. Or we may create stories where we are wronged or hurt. We assume hurtful intentions on the part of the other person. Again, we tell the story over and over, interpreting the other person's behavior as further evidence of his or her wrongdoing. A process referred to as dialoguing helps individuals to clarify their motivations and thoughts to one another and come to a shared understanding of what happened between the two people. In order for this to work, each person must come to the dialogue with an open heart and expectation of deep listening and clear speech. Before dialogue, though, each person must be willing to get in touch with his or her own emotions and motivations. In other words, both need to own or take responsibility for "their own stuff." Being aware of our thoughts and applying the understanding that these thoughts are just stories is the first step to being able to let them go. We learn to see our thoughts as nothing more than creations of the mind. These thought patterns can be broken, however, by bringing mindful awareness to its links to the body. Directly sensing the body in the present moment turns up the volume on the body's messages and turns down the volume on mental chatter. In other words, we "change the channel" from thinking our compulsive thoughts to thinking about something else. One might instead try to recite a favorite poem or sing a favorite song. Likewise, the body scan is a meditation where the individual scans his or her body from toe to head while focusing on the sensations that he or she feels as attention moves from one part of the body to another. Again, the point is both to change what the person is thinking about and ground him or her in the present task of physical sensation.[7]

Finally, meditation can teach the practitioner to be self-compassionate. Psychologist Kristen Neff argues that meditation is more effective when it is combined with self-compassion.[8] Human beings often compare themselves to others, resulting in feelings of inferiority—that they are not wealthy enough, smart enough, thin enough, or good enough. As a consequence, we feel inadequate. We may even feel shame if we are convinced that we do not measure up to others. Some of the women in this study were concerned that they were not attractive enough or young enough now that they were going through menopause. Others felt anxious or out of control. Two said that they felt that they were going mad due, at least in part, to menopause. We can practice self-compassion for ourselves and others with metta (meaning loving-kindness) meditations. Rather than focusing on the breath, the practitioner chants the following silently, first for him or herself and then for all beings:

May I/we be happy.

May I/we be well.

May I/we be free from harm.

May I/we live with ease.

Meditation can be used to make each of us a better person, less reactive, less insistent that things be a certain way. It can also end our suffering, freeing us from compulsive thinking and allowing us to live with things as they are. It can help us to learn more about ourselves and what triggers our negative emotions.[9] It all begins with a curious, open awareness.

FEELING OUT OF CONTROL

A number of women felt out of control during menopause. Kathy said:

I did not know that it would throw my whole body into a frenzy. . . . Before I even knew that they were symptoms of menopause . . . I was a screaming lunatic. Irritability. The people in my life definitely noticed [looking sad]. . . . Fortunately, I could keep my shit together at work, but at home I was a screaming lunatic. . . . I knew I would be better if we weren't home, so we went out *a lot* [her emphasis]. . . . It was frightening because it was an out-of-body experience. I was not the same person I had been. I had no control over my emotions. It seems like it is never ending. There is uncertainty every day. Who is going to wake up? Dr. Jekyll or Mr. Hyde? I was ugly, ugly. . . . By the time I made it through a year with no period, I was more under control than I had been. I had my act together on the inside and outside, too.

Kathy did not try meditation, but she confided that she wished that she had. Kathy had her husband, who is a physician and with whom she could discuss various treatments, as well as her primary care provider. She explained, "He [her husband] would bring home research studies and gave me advice about what to do. He helped to educate me. I trusted his opinion. . . . He didn't leave me which I think is amazing." As the feelings of being out of control grew, Kathy went back to her doctor for antidepressants, which she said helped. Later in the interview she said, "I kind of wish that I had done the meditation. I have found that it is helpful for life in general. I took a year of meditation classes after I went through cancer."

Nina experienced anxiety, depression, and mania when she went through menopause. Her mother also suffered from anxiety at the change of life. Nina said that the anxiety and panic attacks were the most difficult part of menopause for her. She began addressing the symptoms first by seeing an acupuncturist in order to "get stabilized," as she put it. This was the beginning of starting to feel more in control. She also saw an endocrinologist to address thyroid complications and a therapist for the panic attacks that she was experiencing. Nina also took meditation and mindfulness classes and Kundalini yoga classes to learn from her own wisdom. Eventually a nurse practitioner would prescribe a psychotropic medication to get her panic attacks under control. Several years later, at the time of the interview, Nina was again in control of her emotions and her life.

Putting a Spotlight on Denise's Story

Denise's story really began with the birth of her brother, Samuel. Denise's mother, Sue, was a teenage mom. Sue married Sam's father at the age of fifteen, and Sam was born just shy of Sue's sixteenth birthday. Sam's father turned out to be abusive and an alcoholic. Sue and Sam often went hungry and were fearful of the man they lived with. Sam's father beat him when he cried to make him tougher. He abused Sue as well. With no job skills, Sue stayed with her husband until she could take it no longer. Sue returned home to her parents when Sam turned five and sued her husband for divorce. In the 1950s a woman needed to prove abandonment or abuse to get a divorce, so Sue asked a friend to testify to the bruises she had seen on Sue's arms and face. Sue's parents reluctantly agreed to let Sue move back home with Sam, despite the fact that they believed a wife should stay with her husband under all circumstances.

Denise believed that this was the start of her story, because her mother would never develop beyond that scared fifteen-year-old girl. Sue continued to live in fear her whole life and to see life as a "bitch." She would marry Denise's father despite the fact that he treated her like a sex object and controlled her. When Denise asked her mother about it later, Sue replied, "I married your father because I thought you deserved a roof over your head and food on the table." This was the atmosphere in which Denise and Samuel grew up.

Denise's father left her mother when Sue became pregnant. He was convinced that Sue was trying to trap him into marriage. Sue, Denise, and Samuel continued to live with Sue's parents, although it was no place for a teenage boy. Sue's parents were strict and blamed Samuel for Sue's first marriage. Sue and Denise shared a bedroom for the first five years of Denise's life.

Denise's father returned around the time that she turned five. Sue and her children moved into an apartment that Denise's father, Ron, purchased for them. Sue continued to work outside of the home, but they received some of Ron's salary. Ron traveled extensively, and his mother handled his money. Sue would have to ask Ron's mother for money. She had no car, and she and the children walked everywhere they went. In the meantime, Sue's parents were furious that their daughter and granddaughter no longer lived with them.

Denise continued to live with her mother and brother in the apartment that her father rented. Once again, she shared a bedroom with her mother. This time, though, the bedroom was also shared with her father when he returned from traveling. This lasted until Denise turned ten years old. It was upsetting to Denise that she could sometimes hear her parents having sex and that her father walked around in the nude. Denise begged her parents to move to a place where she could have her own room, which they did shortly after Denise turned ten. During this time, Denise's parents married.

Ron's display of his sexuality continued to bother Denise. He would grope her mother in front of Denise and friends of the family. Ron also said obscene things about Denise's maturing body. He even made comments about Sam's girlfriends' bodies. Ron also continued to walk around in the nude in the late evening and night. Denise hated her father and begged her mother to talk to him and get him to wear shorts at night and not say things about Denise's maturing body. Both of her parents ignored her, though, and made no change.

Denise's parents afforded Sam significant latitude in his life. He smoked cigarettes regularly by the time he was in junior high school. Sam quit school by the time he was a sophomore in high school and married in his early twenties. He managed his home life by being gone most of the time. The parents took the exact opposite approach with Denise, though. Unlike Sam, Denise did not have a car and was "stuck" at home until she started college. Denise's mother was absolutely terrified that something would happen to her. Denise explained:

> My mother suffocated me. My cousin visited when I was in high school. We went to a play that was performed at school and then stopped for an ice cream on the way home. My mother acted like we had been out all night. She assumed that the play would get over much earlier than it did and that we would be home at lightning speed. All we did was stop for ice cream. She was pacing back and forth, convinced that we were kidnapped or the car had rolled over in a ditch. My cousin was shocked by my mother, but I was used to her being unreasonable like this. We were home before 10:00 p.m., as teenagers. . . I wasn't really allowed to be a teenager because my mother was so fragile. I had to tiptoe around her or she would get depressed and go deep within herself. Then I would be left all alone. I did not realize it at the time, but I was taking care of her.

Much to her surprise, Denise's father committed suicide soon after she graduated from college. Denise's first thought was that she would now be responsible solely for her mother. Denise felt responsible for keeping her mother from being depressed, which she said was no small feat. Sue was understandably lonely. Denise and her fiancée helped Sue with the chores around Sue's house in the country. There were always things that needed to get done, which was difficult for Denise, given that she lived several states away. Still, she tried to be there for her mother as best as she could.

Throughout Denise's life, she was drawn to her female teachers. Her first memories were of trying to hold her teacher's hand during recess in the first grade. She said that she liked the warm feeling that she got when she held the teacher's hand. Denise hoped that the teacher would take her home. She continued to be drawn to teachers throughout high school and college. They provided role models for her to escape from the life that she had with her parents. She hoped that one of her teachers would take her to live with them someday. However, this caused problematic relationships with her teachers, although some were more compassionate and under-standing than others. Denise said that she did eventually become friends with one of her college professors, who invited her into her personal life and served as a mentor for her.

Denise said that she fell apart after her father died. She and her then-husband were both in graduate school, which was a very pressured environment for both. Denise was trying to help her mother as much as possible but was not able to "fix" her mother's loneliness or financial prob-lems. Denise knew that Sue thought she should do more for her, Sue, but Denise needed space between her and her mother and grandparents. It became a struggle for much of Denise's adulthood.

For the first years of Denise's marriage, she would beat her chest in frustration and rage. It was not until after menopause and three years of therapy and meditation that Denise realized that the frustration and rage were due to her parents not seeing her as separate from them, with her own needs and desire for self-development. Denise's mother and grandparents were dependent on her for their own self-fulfillment and did not realize "where they ended and [she] began," as she explained it. Denise was unaware of all this, though, when she began perimenopause. She explained:

> I felt totally out of control at the start of menopause. I had been a very together, organized professional. By then, though, I felt like I had ADD, always jumping from one thing to another. I did things that were not a part of my personality. I went bungee jumping and got a nose ring. I took up water skiing. Mostly, though, I just felt really agitated and out of control. I would burn everything I cooked because I forgot about things in the oven. I was just a mess.

Denise went to see her gynecologist for HRT. Her gyn said that it was too late for her to start HRT because her FSH levels were already high. Denise's doctor said that she would have suggested a SNRI except that Denise was already taking one. Denise also started seeing a therapist. Denise said that it was then that "the shit hit the fan."

Denise started seeing her therapist in the first year or two of perimeno-pause. She said that she felt extremely angry and was having difficulty getting along with people. She particularly resented her mother's visits, although she felt somewhat distant from her husband as well. Denise added:

> It was then that I started feeling attached to my female therapist like I had with my female teachers for all those years. I of course told my therapist about it, about the fact that I felt connected to her. She told me that it wasn't possible for us to be friends, because she was my therapist, and that I had to let it go. But I couldn't. I knew that it was crazy, but I needed her to be in my life, to feel whole. . . . It was then that I read about meditation as a way of creating new neural pathways in the brain. I thought maybe I could rewire my brain to be less negative. It was the start of changing my life.

Denise turned to meditation and a new therapist who would help her to understand the impact of her history on her life. Denise said that it took time to see the effects of meditation and therapy. Her therapist helped her to recognize her frustration with her mother and the way that their lives had been enmeshed. Denise began to realize how unhealthy their relationship had been and how abandoned she had felt when her mother had not been there for her. Sue had not recognized Denise's needs when her father behaved inappropriately around her and when her father died. She had not thought about the fact that Denise had lost her father, only that she herself had lost her husband. The therapist helped Denise realize that she had always taken care of her mother from infancy onward. She had taken care of her mother so that her mother could take care of her, except that her mother often had not taken care of her.

This was where meditation played a key role in Denise's healing. It was meditation that first alerted her to her unmet needs. Denise felt her own anger when going through the body scan meditation. She also realized that she felt empty in her stomach and disconnected from the others in her family. Denise would eventually learn to visualize her mother being on her own and setting boundaries around her own being. She understood that she had turned to her teachers as a way of being seen and of having someone strong who could be there for her, despite the fact that it had never been realized. Denise recognized that her rage, which she had expressed by beating her chest, was the result of her parents ignoring her needs and going about being inattentive to the psychological needs of a teenager. Denise added:

The biggest thing that I gained from meditation and mindfulness, though, was the ability to let it go, to let things be as they are. I have always tried to change my mother so that she could be there for me. I thought I needed her, but I don't. What she does, what mistakes she makes, has no impact on me. I can still go about my own life and not get caught up in her needs. I can set boundaries, and that is not selfish. I have learned that I cannot fix my mother, but I am able to be more compassionate than I was in the past. I can be more compassionate since I don't need her to be there for me. It is so liberating! It is like we have become unmeshed, and I can be on my own now even though she would prefer that we were still enmeshed.

Denise said that she still continues her meditation and mindfulness practice. She has to be aware of when she is feeling isolated and to reach out to her friends to prevent depression. Denise is no longer on an SNRI and is no longer seeing a therapist. She also recites a loving-kindness meditation, or metta, that goes thus: "May all beings be free from harm. May all beings be free from suffering. May all beings be happy. May all beings be at ease." She said that it has helped her to forgive her parents because she now understands that they, too, were the products of their own circumstances and conditions. Denise believes that menopause was a godsend because it brought her to therapy and meditation, both of which have brought her to a place of acceptance and relaxation for the first time in her life.

CONCLUSION

Meditation provides opportunities in many different ways to address feelings of anger and being out of control, which frequently come up during menopause. It can also be used to help women to address unresolved conflict or emotions from their past or to accept the things that they cannot change.

During meditation, the amygdala, the site of the flight-or-fright response, is dampened while the frontal lobe is activated, allowing women to work through their emotions. By paying attention to all the thoughts that come up in their minds, women can become more aware of the things that are bothering them. However, they can also allow those emotions to pass by them by exercising the Buddhist principle that "all things shall pass" (including our thoughts and emotions) because change is constant. Likewise, our thoughts are nothing more than the manifestations of our mind, often without the truth that we attribute to them out of our own desire to protect ourselves. Recognizing the possibility that our own perspective of events with others in our lives may be faulty also provides room for the possibility that we have been wrong and allows us to open up dialogue with those with whom we have been in conflict.

The practice of meditation teaches us to accept things as they are in the present. This includes physical and emotional discomfort and pain, making it easier for the practitioner to manage the symptoms of menopause such as hot flashes and feeling out of control. It allows women to pause before expressing angry feelings that arise in menopause. By paying greater attention to our thoughts, we can become aware of compulsive thinking and liberate ourselves from its clutches. We can become more aware of destructive triggers that send us to false refuges that may bring only shame or greater clinging to negative coping mechanisms. It can also make us more aware of the ways we shield ourselves from the painful parts of our lives because they frighten us. We put up barriers based on our opinions and prejudices, and we cling to the belief that only we are in the right. Only by being at one with our suffering and living in the here and now with an acceptance of things as they are will we be able to free ourselves from these destructive habits. While we learn to do this, it behooves us all to treat ourselves with loving-kindness. Things are always changing, but we can live with change and uncertainty, like that experienced during menopause, as long as we accept things as they are.

Meditation and mindfulness, then, help women to not only manage the symptoms of menopause and the emotions that arise with it but also to come out on the other side of menopause as a healthier person with far greater resilience and adaptability. Women who practice meditation during menopause have the potential not only to resolve prior conflict in their lives and to work with painful emotions from the past but also to be able to live with uncertainty and change and to avoid the false refuges that entice so many of us. It is the beginning of our own awakening and liberation.

Examples of women utilizing meditation to various extents were discussed. Kathy did not try meditation during menopause, although she wished that she had. She did, however, successfully try it after undergoing treatment for cancer. Nina was able to feel in greater control with the assistance of a variety of methods, including meditation, mindfulness, yoga, and acupuncture. Nina also relied on psychotropic medication and therapy as well. Denise used meditation and mindfulness most extensively, proclaiming that it changed her life for the better and that she came out of menopause feeling much stronger and more spiritually developed as a result of all that she learned through meditation.

NINE

Conclusion

There were multiple objectives for this book. One of the goals was to examine the range of women's menopausal experiences. There is no typical experience that all women share from one class or race or even family. Women's situations vary considerably. Our own individual experiences are a sum of where we fall on the range of various symptoms and treatments along with variations in timing and severity of those symptoms. The women in this book started menopause as early as thirty-eight years of age, although all were at least perimenopausal by the age of fifty-two. Likewise, the length of perimenopause ranged from being nonexistent to lasting eight years. That is, some women experienced menopausal symptoms for eight years before entering the last year in which they had no period. For many women, the symptoms in perimenopause were more painful than those in the last year of menopause. Women more often stopped menstruating several times before they would go without a period for one full year, which is referred to as a "false start" to the last year. Many also had lingering symptoms after menopause ended, although the symptoms occurred less often and were less intense than they had been during perimenopause and menopause.

Women sought different treatments, dependent in part on the severity of the symptoms and the social meaning they attributed to menopause. Women with the most severe symptoms pursued HRT. One woman sought HRT even before her symptoms began though because she did not want the inconvenience of menopause and because she associated menopause with feeling out of control, which frightened her. Some women requested hormone replacement, but their physicians told them that their symptoms were not severe enough to warrant HRT. Physicians are typically reluctant to prescribe hormone replacement (a combination of estrogen and progestin) because of the increased likelihood of breast cancer, among other health problems.[1,2] Physicians instead prescribe SSRIs or SNRIs to treat symptoms as they moderate body temperature fluctuations and reduce anxiety and depression.[3] Although not as effective as HRT, they have been found to at least reduce the severity of the symptoms. Likewise, phytoestrogens and bioidentical hormones are also suggested to alleviate symptoms. Bioidentical hormones are most often used to treat vaginal dryness and come in the form of ointments and vaginal rings.[4] Soy products are a commonly used source of phytoestrogens. Likewise, women can purchase supplements on the internet that contain a number of phytoestrogens.[5] Only a few of the women sought these treatments, although they were not as well known as HRT, which was widely publicized before being found to cause breast cancer. Most women knew that exercise and reducing caffeine and alcohol would help alleviate symptoms of menopause and that vitamin D and calcium supplements would reduce the likelihood of osteoporosis.

Despite the variation, we can still draw some generalizations based on women's experiences. For example, there was a tendency to look for a pharmacological solution to the symptoms of menopause regardless of defining menopause as a natural occurrence. Perhaps we persist in looking in that direction because the most effective treatment to date has been a pharmacological one. Westerners expect medicine to alleviate discomfort, especially if it becomes debilitating. One of the women said that she is confident that the pharmaceutical industry will develop a product that is as effective as hormone replacement but will be safer than HRT. This suggests though that menopause continues to be partly medicalized in that we continue to seek a medical solution. Women request HRT far more often than it is prescribed. However, younger generations are looking more toward Eastern practices such as acupuncture, yoga, and meditation to alleviate the symptoms of menopause. There is evidence that although meditation does not reduce the severity of hot flashes, it does allow women to manage their symptoms better.[6] Likewise, women can use mindfulness to take advantage of changes in the brain during menopause and address unresolved conflict or consider new directions in life. Dr. Christiane Northrup argues that the need to address these issues is highlighted at menopause when our lives and emotions are put under a microscope.[7] In sum, at least some younger women have moved from defining menopause as a medical problem to be treated with a pharmacological intervention to seeing it as a natural part of the life course that can be best addressed with changes in lifestyle, such as diet and exercise, and a psychospiritual perspective. However, there is still some continuation of the medicalization of menopause or the expectation that we should pursue pharmacological solutions to treat the loss of estrogen. This is due, in part, to the media's portrayal of menopause as a physical deficit that should be eliminated and the medical community's predominance in earlier treatments.[8]

THE SOCIAL MEANING OF MENOPAUSE

The social construction or meaning of menopause comes in part from a woman's place in the social structure of society, including her level of education, race, and class, and the historical time period. Many of the women had a negative view of menopause. The symptoms of menopause were often much worse than they expected them to be, resulting in an overall unfavorable meaning associated with menopause. What was far more difficult, though, was that some women viewed menopause as ruining their lives because they could no longer bear children and were afraid that they would no longer be as sexually appealing or as attractive as they once were. One of the women stated that she recognized that it was sad that she saw menopause this way, but it did not change how she viewed it. Yet, none of these women had any intention of having more children when they went through menopause. They had not completed college and worked in part-time jobs while their husbands worked full time. Living in a male-dominated family culture left them feeling a loss of status in later life. They saw fewer options for meaningful roles in the second half of life that could sustain their status and self-worth.

This is in contrast to the results of a study of older women by Heather Dillaway. The women in this study saw menopause as a "good" aspect of getting older. These women were comparing menopause to other aspects of aging. In that context, they saw menopause more positively. They pointed out that they enjoyed sex more upon menopause. The women in Dillaway's study were older and aware of just how difficult other aspects of aging can be.[9] In addition, menopause and other life course events may be seen more positively the further we are from the event. Winterich argues that menopause has been constructed by clinical communities and popular culture as a solely biological or physiological event and a negative

period of loss. She further points out that individual women find menopause to be an inconsequential or positive experience overall.[10] That was
not the case in this study, however. The women here were more likely to
share their negative experiences, in part because they were closer to them
due to being younger than the women in Winterich's study and because
their symptoms were so severe. Their experiences were worse than what
they expected, perhaps because older women told them that their own
experiences were inconsequential or even positive. The women in this
study were also closer to losing their reproductive roles and their status
associated with their sexual appeal. This was a particularly difficult loss
for women with less education.

African American women were far less likely to seek medical assistance as a result of their construction of menopause. They defined menopause within an overall distrust of the medical community because of a
history of physicians encouraging unnecessary hysterectomies and using
African Americans disproportionately in medical trials or experiments.[11,12]
African Americans said that their friends and family encouraged them to
avoid going to a doctor despite a high rate of fibroids among African
American women. However, African American women were less likely to
talk about the severity of their symptoms or go into detail on every symptom they experienced. They seemed to have a more positive view of menopause, in part because they wished to distance themselves from white
women, whom they saw as unable to endure hardship. African American
women may also attribute more positive meaning to menopause because
of their continued status as the matriarchs of their families following
menopause.

Latina women fell into two groups, with disparate reactions to menopause. Some of the women took a very combative approach, making it
clear that they would not allow menopause to bother them the way that it
did white women. They also pointed to the fact that their families depended
on them, so they could not allow menopause to disrupt their lives. Other
Latina women felt that they should just allow menopause to occur as it
does naturally. They tended not to talk with others about menopause or
seek support or treatment. If anything, they seemed to be embarrassed by
being menopausal. Women may not want others to know their age because
of the importance of their youth and attractiveness in a machismo
culture.

A minority of women saw menopause in a very positive light. They
were overjoyed by no longer having a period or being worried about

pregnancy. They saw a number of opportunities that were now open to them in later life that were not options before. Their children no longer needed as much supervision and were no longer living at home. This gave the women much greater freedom to pursue new interests or devote more time to things they wished to do. Women believed that they could consider a new career if they wished, because they no longer had to make as much money as they once did. More importantly, they stated that they no longer felt that they had to "prove themselves" or pursue high-status jobs. Neither did they feel it necessary any longer to follow appropriate societal norms like entertaining in their homes. Overall, they saw menopause as a very joyous and liberating time in their lives.

Most of the women viewed menopause as being a mix of positive and negative aspects. Overwhelmingly, they said that the downside was that menopause meant that they were now old or aging. However, these women will have more years of postmenopausal life where they are disease-free than any previous generation. Today's elders can expect to live half of their adult lives postmenopause. In addition, they are more similar to younger generations in terms of health and physical ability than ever before. To the women, though, aging was an overall negative thing. They did note the fact that they no longer had to manage the pain and inconvenience of menstruating, and a few mentioned a better sex life. More of the women who had difficult periods saw menopause as very positive or a mixed positive and negative experience.

EASTERN INFLUENCES

Some of the younger women looked toward Eastern practices in their treatment of menopause. This included use of acupuncture, yoga, meditation, and mindfulness. Women sought acupuncture to balance their hormones and the systems in their bodies in general. There is some indication that the targeting of pressure points or energy channels can lower the rate of hot flashes by as much as 35 percent.[13] Acupuncture is also said to decrease insomnia, night sweats, mood imbalance, fatigue, and general pain. Only a few women sought acupuncture for menopause, however.

A minority of women also turned to yoga and meditation or mindfulness for menopause. They explained that yoga made them feel better in general and helped them to be more flexible. Meditation and being mindful also increased their overall well-being and helped them to manage their hot flashes and other symptoms better than they had before.[14] Meditation and mindfulness also helped women to recognize changes that they wanted to make in their lives and to tackle unresolved conflict. New information about how the brain changes at menopause and how meditation can be used to alter patterns in the brain clarify just how these Eastern practices, along with talk therapy, can be beneficial for women during menopause and may explain why younger generations of women are turning to these practices at menopause.[15,16,17,18]

The movement to evaluate one's priorities and focus on unresolved conflict is part of a trend toward greater self-actualization in younger generations of menopausal or postmenopausal women. These are the same women who participated in higher rates of divorce in the 1970s and 1980s when they found their marriages to be less than fulfilling. People expect more from life than previous generations did. As such, they are more willing to pursue meditation to awaken their best selves and optimize the remaining years of their lives. The need to do so is even more important now that postmenopausal women have half of their adult lives still before them.

Women who meditated noticed thoughts about unresolved conflict in their marriages and relationships with other family members. They noticed a desire to change their careers or cut back on their work hours. Others noticed fears of loss, depression, and problematic relationships from their childhoods. Meditation allows the practitioner to notice an emotion and to be with it completely before letting the emotion go rather than clinging to it. Meditation also activates the frontal lobe of the brain. The frontal lobe is what allows the practitioner to work through emotions and to have access to the emotional landscape from which he or she can respond. Meditation also causes the amygdala, where the fight or flight automatic response gets triggered, to calm down, making it possible to avoid a quick reaction and to process the emotion instead. Meditation improves the well-being of women overall during menopause.

The practice of meditation also encourages the practitioner to live in the present rather than ruminating about the past or longing for a better future, which may or may not result. It inspires the acceptance of things as they are rather than trying to create perfect conditions that may not occur. As such, women who meditate can live more effectively with change and uncertainty, such as occurs with menopause. Buddhism reminds us that our thoughts are not necessarily truths, despite the fact that we are constantly telling ourselves stories about events that have occurred that verify that we are in the right. This knowledge makes it more likely that we will consider alternative understandings of events and be open to the possibility of misunderstandings. It helps us to recognize compulsive thinking and how to let it go. It also makes us aware of destructive thoughts or triggers that send us to false refuges out of fear of the painful parts of our lives. Meditation inspires us to pull down the barriers we erect to shield ourselves, such as our opinions and prejudices. In short, meditation allows us to live with greater liberation and well-being and with far less suffering throughout life.

SYMPTOMOLOGY

The results of this research highlight women's desire to control their symptoms. This is especially true for white women, who were far more likely to seek treatment from physicians than were African American or Latina women. This is also evidenced by the abundance of products online and on the market in general that are designed to alleviate symptoms. Each claims to do so "naturally" but offers little or no evidence of effectiveness. The media in general focuses on the symptoms of menopause while making light of those symptoms or using humor to discuss them. A good example of this is *Menopause The Musical*, which helps women to poke fun at their experiences while simultaneously normalizing them. Much of our construction of menopause or the meaning we give to menopause is framed by the difficulty of its symptoms and its biophysiological foundation rather than looking at the opportunities that come from menopause or looking at menopause as a life course event.

Many of the women pointed out that menopause resulted in an improvement in their marriages and/or sex lives. Menopause highlighted any need for change in their marriage or any unresolved conflict. Menopause also gave their husbands an opportunity to be helpful or supportive during the process, and some were. Likewise, some of the women thought that their libido was higher once they were off birth control pills and no longer had to spend long hours in child-rearing. However, these positive factors did not come out in their construction of menopause nearly as much as their focus on symptoms.

MALE MENOPAUSE

Early on in this research, the author was asked why she did not include male menopause in the study. What is sometimes referred to as male menopause, or andropause, however, is quite different from female menopause. In fact, it is not clear whether male menopause is a myth or not. It is most commonly thought of as nothing more than a normal part of aging in men, rather than a separate life course event. The change in sex hormones occurs much more gradually in men than it does in women. There is a moderate decrease in levels of testosterone of 1 percent in men starting at around thirty years old.[19] Although low testosterone is significantly related to a decrease in sex drive and erectile dysfunction, it has only a weak association with other physical and/or psychological symptoms. Male menopause does not cause dramatic symptoms like night sweats or hot flashes that are characteristic signs of menopause for women. A study in the *New England Journal of Medicine* suggests that only 2 percent of men experience andropause, whereas all women go through menopause (i.e., they eventually stop menstruating) if they live long enough.

Both situations, however, point to the need to modify the social construction of masculinity and femininity. Masculinity is defined most commonly by high levels of testosterone, strength (both physical and psychological), and power. At its most toxic level, it can lead to violence, an inability to show emotion, and an unhealthy obsession with body building and highly competitive and damaging sports such as football and boxing. In defining it this way, we leave some older men feeling less than masculine, possibly leading to low self-esteem and depression in old age. We leave men of all ages being unable to feel masculine if they do not play football, drink heavily, or live a high-risk lifestyle. We also need to move away from a gendered construction of femininity that is defined exclusively by reproduction, youth, and attractiveness. We need to instead value the roles of older women and the characteristics that they embody. As we have seen, there are many vital contributions that postmenopausal women provide and important roles that they assume in society and in the family. It is physically detrimental and psychologically damaging for women to dread menopause because they can no longer bear children or no longer have an hourglass figure. There is much more to femininity and the female experience than this narrow construction.

"MY HORMONES DON'T CONTROL ME"

Women who had not yet started menopause believed that they would be able to control their symptoms with over-the-counter products. One woman went so far as to say, "I don't allow my hormones to control me or affect my behavior." Such a statement reflects second-wave feminism, which denies innate differences between men and women. Second-wave feminism lost sight of the benefits of gender differences and the fact that difference does not have to mean inequality.

The women in this study would take issue with a statement that suggests they could control their hot flashes, night sweats, insomnia, and other symptoms. They would be offended by Friedan's assumption that society overinflates what can be debilitating symptoms of menopause. Though not all women experience menopause negatively, there are many who do. We do them a disservice when we turn a blind eye to their lived experiences. Recognizing our hormones and their impact does not mean that we are defined or confined by our biology. Failing to recognize them does, however, deny women the legitimacy of their experience and the potential of finding a safe, effective alternative to HRT.

Younger women to whom I spoke assume that there are "natural products" that alleviate menopausal symptoms. They believe that they will not be inconvenienced by menopause because of these natural products. There is no treatment that is as effective as HRT in treating menopausal symptoms. This statement cannot be emphasized enough. Symptoms can continue past menopause for some women, even when they remain on HRT. What is true, however, is that many women find some relief from symptoms using nonhormonal treatments and that HRT can be effective at very low doses and for short periods.

What I hope women have learned from this book is that they are not alone, no matter what their menopausal experience is like. There is a wide range of menopause experiences, with some women having severe symptoms and others waking up to find that they have gone through menopause asymptomatically. The fact that men and women are affected by their hormones does not make either one a victim. Hormonal effects require treatment, but it is available and still under development. To assume otherwise may prevent that development, leave women feeling that there must be something wrong with them, and deny the differences between men and women.

Still, we must fight the limited constructions of masculinity and femininity that equate men with testosterone and women with their reproductive capacity. Each deprives us of all that is open to us in the second half of life when testosterone and estrogen begin to wane. There are many roles that are open after midlife to women that cannot be fulfilled by younger women. Older women greatly improve our society, as do older men. It is time that we value their roles and contributions.

More importantly, it is time we recognize the disservice we do to women going through menopause when we lead them to believe that their lives are over because they are no longer capable of having children. It has been a long time since we needed to encourage reproduction to populate the United States. Women cannot and should not try to maintain the same body weight and shape they had in high school. We need to do a better job in recognizing the difficulties of menopause and supporting women through it rather than underplaying the experience out of fear that it will hold women back in a male-oriented world. Women do not have to be like men. We need not neglect their experiences and undermine them out of fear that feminism will lose the ground that it has made. We are past this, and it is time we recognized it.

The results of this research are also a wake-up call to the medical community that African American women are afraid to see a doctor, especially a gynecologist, out of fear of unnecessary hysterectomies. In fact, African American women need to see their gynecologists more than white women because of higher rates of fibroids, which can lead to complications. Yet, while white women complained that they could not get a hysterectomy when they wanted one because physicians were afraid that they would change their minds and want a child later, black women believed that they would be given a hysterectomy without their consent. This is not surprising, given the medical community's history of using black men and women for medical experiments. Clearly the medical community needs to increase its racial sensitivity to black women and assure them that nothing will be done without their consent and that they will not be pushed into having a procedure that they do not want. While medical schools contend that they have enhanced their programs to the benefit of the doctor-patient relationship, they have not done enough for all patients, such as marginalized African American women. It is time to change that.

It is possible for menopause to be the start of a joyous time in women's lives, although it is clearly not all smooth sailing. By knowing oneself better through the trials of menopause and the benefits of meditation and mindfulness, women can come out of the experience with an enhanced sense of well-being. Through addressing their unmet needs of the past, they can lead an improved second half of adulthood. And it all begins with a pause.

APPENDIX A

Glossary of Menopause-Related Terminology

Bioidentical hormones: Bioidentical hormones are used to treat menopausal symptoms and are considered to be safer than synthetic hormones because they have the same structure as our natural hormones. They are synthesized from natural products such as plants to produce the identical structure of hormones as they occur in the body. They are often used to treat vaginal dryness; the vaginal ring Estring™ contains bioidentical hormones.

Estrogen: A hormone produced in the ovaries that is responsible for the development and maintenance of female characteristics, estrogen is also responsible for the regulation of the menstrual cycle and reproductive system. Estrogen levels change at perimenopause. It includes three estrogenic compounds produced naturally in the body: estradiol, estrone, and estriol.

FSH (follicle-stimulating hormone): This hormone, produced by the pituitary gland, stimulates ovulation monthly; physicians test for onset of menopause by measuring the level of FSH in the blood. As ovulation gradually ceases, FSH levels gradually increase; FSH levels remain elevated, causing the changes in the brain during menopause.

GnRH (gonadotropin-releasing hormone): This hormone is produced by the hypothalamus and is responsible for releasing FSH and LH from the pituitary gland; during perimenopause, levels of GnRH rise in the brain causing FSH and LH to surge and stay at elevated levels. Changing levels of GnRH and other hormones prime the brain for new perceptions and new behaviors.

Hormone replacement therapy (HRT): This treatment is no longer encouraged in less severe cases of hot flashes and other symptoms because it increases the likelihood of breast cancer and other conditions; these hormones are referred to as synthetic hormones and include Premarin™, Provera™, and Prempro™. Most birth control pills are a type of synthetic hormone. The term "hormone replacement therapy" is preferred to estrogen replacement therapy because the pills contain progesterone as well as estrogen.

LH (luteinizing hormone): This is a reproductive hormone similar to FSH: levels of LH rise significantly during menopause and are responsible for changes in the brain during this time.

Limbic system: This system is responsible for regulating emotions, behaviors, and motivations; some of these behaviors include ones we need to survive (fight-or-flight response, caring for young, and reproduction).

Menopause: This is the time in a woman's life when menstrual periods stop, and the woman is no longer able to have children; it is operationalized by going without a period for an entire year. Menopause is characterized by low levels of estrogen.

Perimenopause: This is the start of the menopause process when symptoms are often more severe; symptoms may include hot flashes, night sweats, mood swings, irritability, irregular and/or severe periods, weight gain, memory loss, and migraines. There is an imbalance in female hormones caused by the decline of progesterone, resulting in estrogen dominance.

Phytoestrogens: Found in some plants and foods, they help your body adapt to its current hormone level and are therefore used to treat some menopausal symptoms, such as hot flashes and night sweats. Phytoestrogens include isoflavones (this type of phytoestrogen is found in some foods such as soy) and lignans (phytoestrogens found in grain such as flaxseed, fruits, and vegetables) as well as the phytoestrogens found in herbs such as mint, red clover, ginseng, and fennel.

Postmenopause: This is the time after a woman has gone an entire year without a period.

Premenopause: This is the period in a woman's life prior to perimenopause.

Progesterone: This is another hormone produced primarily in the ovaries; it, too, plays a role in reproduction: progesterone prepares the lining of the uterus for the implantation and growth of the embryo. A decline in progesterone is the first hormonal change to cause symptoms in a woman who is beginning perimenopause.

Temporal lobe: This is the site of enhanced intuition; an imbalance in the levels of estrogen versus progesterone "sets the temporal lobe on fire," enhancing women's intuition.

APPENDIX B

Meditations for Working with Difficult Emotions

I attended this workshop, taught by Reverend Steve Kanji Ruhl, on how to use meditation and mindfulness to manage difficult emotions like grief, anger, self-judgment, anxiety, guilt, and shame.[1] Often people escape these emotions through shopping, the internet, and alcohol and other addictions. This workshop helps individuals to engage their emotions in a way that can transform them or let them go.

An emotion is a feeling with a thought attached to it. All emotions have the potential to be painful or difficult—even love, if you cling to it.

Conversely, difficult emotions do not have to be painful if you feel the energy but let the story behind it go. In other words, an emotion can cease to be difficult if you recognize it and accept it without judgment and let it flow through you.

Happiness is something that we all search for, but it is conditional on certain circumstances. Likewise, nothing is permanent and conditions are always changing. As a result, happiness is fleeting.

Joy is not conditional. It is always available, but you must be present to experience it in the here and now.

"This too shall pass" is a Buddhist philosophy. It helps to deal with difficult emotions if you remember that nothing is permanent.

There is always suffering. One source of our suffering is comparing ourselves to others and competing with them. We are better off living simply and not striving for material goods.

Suffering also comes when we resist our emotions. By "stuffing our emotions down," we cause them to become stronger and explode at times that we do not expect.

We need to be aware of our own "issues" and the impact that events may have on our lives, and we need to be aware of creating the "stuff" or "issues" that we carry around with us. Clinging to our beliefs or to our need for things to be a certain way also causes suffering.

Another core belief in Buddhism is the importance of "not knowing." We do not know in most situations. If we can be open to the fact that we do not know something, we will not be as likely to get angry or jump to conclusions. For example, I do not know why someone did not invite me to his or her party. I may assume that I do know that the person did it because he or she does not like me. That would make me sad or angry. It is better to recognize that we do not always know.

Likewise, there is the Buddhist principle on the importance of being, not doing. We love people for who they are, not what they do. You are good for your being, not for your doing. It is enough to be.

"Shadow" is the unconscious material that we repress or deny. This is a Jungian concept. That emotion will eventually erupt in different ways. It will demand to be seen. Difficult emotions are often pushed into the shadow realm. It amplifies their power. The root source of the emotion often gets repressed. The more emotions are repressed, the more powerful they become, and the more that they will come to the surface unexpectedly.

We need to bring our emotions to the surface. Meditation helps us to do that by helping us to recognize them.

Shadow material often gets projected onto others. Being present with the emotion rather than projecting it onto others is the purpose of meditation. Meditation allows us to notice the anger, to look into the source of it, and to be present with it. It allows us to move the emotion out of the shadow realm.

Depression may be due to repressed anger. The anger comes out of fear of something, which is the result of being hurt. The depression may be the manifestation of the anger and other repressed emotions in the shadow realm.

Depression is often caused by underlying anger. What makes us angry is often fear of being hurt. We can address depression by being aware of our fear of being hurt and investigating its source in our lives.

Manifestations of stress and anxiety might include tightening in the chest, a racing heart, and a heightened sense of alertness that is narrowly focused. Meditation can bring that anxiety down. There is acute anxiety when we focus on the story line.

In meditation practice, we are present and can notice that what caused the hurt before is here again. We see that our old ways are showing up again. We might even foreshadow what is going to happen in the future based on our past. Meditation allows us to work through this and to stop the progression to feeling hurt.

Sunyata refers to the principle that all phenomena are empty of inherent substance. Everything in the universe is empty of substance, and nothing is permanent. Therefore, there is nothing that we can really cling to.

We are like the weather, a constantly changing range of emotions that we call the self. The self is a constantly moving back and forth of energies. When the ego self is set aside, one can directly experience what is arising at any moment.

Stressors are relative. Not everyone is stressed by the same thing or anxious because of the same thing. They are relative because they are inherently empty. Therefore, we have choice.

There is a tendency to want to power through these difficult emotions, make oneself numb, or put up a wall of resistance. We can also ignore our difficult emotions by studying them instead of dealing with them or accepting them, or by repressing them.

How, then, do you find well-being in the presence of this shadow or stressor?

Spiritual bypass relies on spiritual practices to avoid our own psychological issues. It is a facade of spiritual correctness without addressing our shadow material or getting psychological treatment. It refers to thinking that if you just meditate enough, you won't have to address your own psychological stuff.

Having loving connections with nature can help us to get away from stress and anxiety. Gratitude and prayer are also effective.

Someone who has experienced severe trauma probably should not meditate before undergoing therapeutic techniques with a trained therapist.

MEDITATION PRACTICES FOR DEALING WITH DIFFICULT EMOTIONS

Shikantaza ("Just Sitting")

This is similar to vipassana or insight meditation. It refers to being completely with the emotion and then letting go of the emotion. It is a way of relinquishing the wall of resistance. The meditation allows you to notice the emotion and be completely with it. You allow it to flow through you rather than cling to it. There is no goal except to be aware of the thoughts that come and go.

Sit on a comfortable cushion, palms up, resting loosely on your knees. You should be sitting erect, as if there is a rod that goes from the top of your head to the bottom of your spine.

Breathe inward and then outward deeply, allowing your breath to flow through you. Concentrate on your breath. You will inevitably have thoughts that interrupt your concentration on the breath. Notice them and gently return to concentrating on your breath. There is no way to do it wrong. When you realize that you are thinking of something else, just return to your breath. Notice what you are thinking and what sensations you are experiencing.

It has been shown that meditation activates the frontal lobe of the brain. The frontal lobe is what allows you to work through emotions and to have access to your emotional landscape. Meditation also causes the amygdala to calm down. The amygdala is where the fight-or-flight response gets triggered. Meditation then makes it possible to avoid a quick reaction and to process the emotion instead. Shikantaza allows you to be completely with the emotion and then let it go.

Being totally present with the stress or anxiety is the only way to go to a place without it. It is the only way to get away from the story line and to stop clinging to the self.

The value of shikantaza is to be aware of all the thoughts that come and go, instead of pushing the emotions away. Again, it is being with the emotion and then letting it go.

Visualizing one's emotions and thoughts is a function of the practice, not a goal. You sit with your emotions rather than pushing them away. By being one with them, you can get away from them. They are no longer repressed and able to explode.

Council Circle

This is a useful exercise for dyads, particularly when there is a power differential. The goal is for each person to speak from the heart and listen from the heart. It creates an environment where difficult emotions can be addressed. It could be used in family therapy. The key is that as long as someone holds the *talking piece*, he or she cannot be interrupted. The others in the circle should be listening without judgment. Also, there is no cross-talk. You do not address the other person. Anything said in the Council Circle is confidential. It is a safe space. It is useful for discussing sources of stress and anxiety. Each person should speak of what is coming from the heart at that time.

Place comfortable chairs in a circle so that individuals are looking at one another. In the middle of the circle, place a "talking piece." It can be any object, such as a stick. The intention is that anyone who picks up the talking piece and holds it can speak without being interrupted while the others in the circle are expected to listen with an open mind. Allow each person to speak, and leave time at the end for anyone who wants to speak a second or third time.

The Body-Mind Scan

This guided meditation was developed by Jon Kabat-Zinn and is particularly effective for treating stress and anxiety, as well as other difficult emotions.

The person lies on his or her back with the palms up. The guide has the person focus on each part of his or her body, one at a time, beginning with the toes and going up through the top of the head. The guide tells the person to breathe in relaxation and breathe out stress and anxiety at each body part. The person is asked to feel what sensations are present and to notice them. It helps him or her both to relax and to be aware of anxieties or thoughts that come up as he or she scans through the body.

R.A.I.N.

The R.A.I.N. exercise was developed by Tara Brach.[2] It is particularly effective for managing feelings of shame, self-judgment, and guilt. The Dalai Lama could not understand that people may not love themselves. We do not value just "being." We only value "doing." Mr. Rogers taught children the importance of their just being and valuing themselves or who they are. There is unconditional love for just being.

If we can get through all the layers of our "stuff" and the shadow material, we can get to our inherent perfection. We are enlightened and perfect by our very nature of being. We hope to awaken people to see their own inherent, awakened being. We meditate because we are awakened.

R.A.I.N. is a guided meditation for self-compassion. Tara Brach recently adapted it from Buddhism.

RECOGNIZE: What is this thing that is making you feel bad about your-self? What is missing? What is making you feel empty or has put you into a trance? Recognize the emotion and name it.

ALLOW (or ACCEPT): Where do you feel this emotion? Allow your feel-ings to be just as they are. Experience the swelling of deep grief and whisper, "This too," or "I consent." Allow the feeling to be without pushing it away. Just by whispering a phrase like "I consent," you loosen the resistance and allow yourself to be one with the emotion.

INVESTIGATE: Investigate the emotion. Where do you feel this? Is it sharp or dull? What does the emotion feel like in the mind and body? Ask yourself what you need to heal. What do you need right now?

NURTURE: Ask yourself what you would be if you stopped judging your-self or being afraid or feeling shame or guilt. What would it be like if you were no longer at war with yourself? Give yourself what you found you need under "Investigate." Maybe what you need is to say "It is okay." Maybe it is to say "I love you."

Loving-Kindness Meditation

A loving-kindness meditation is useful for working with anger, fear, and grief. Anger is considered to be one of the three poisons. However, anger can also have positive qualities. You can transfer the energy into something more useful like righteous indignation. Anger can also help you to see the issue that needs to be addressed.

Fear has an element of hyperawareness. It can be transformed into being aware of what is present. Likewise, the energy of grief has a quality of love that we can access. If we resist these energies, they will grow stronger. We need to rechannel the energies into allies.

The practitioner sits on a comfortable cushion and closes his or her eyes. The practitioner is asked to imagine a loved one. He or she then chants to that person: "May you be happy. May you be well. May you be free from harm." Then the practitioner does the same thing for a neutral person, someone he or she neither loves nor dislikes. He or she then does the same thing for someone whom he or she considers an enemy or for whom he or she holds difficult emotions. The practitioner then chants the same three sentences for him- or herself.

This is a technique to turn anger around and open up the heart. By expressing the loving-kindness to oneself after one's enemy, the practitioner can see the connection between oneself and one's enemy.

Similar to this is the practice of tonglen, where the practitioner breathes in the pain and suffering of others and then breathes out love and compassion.[3]

Feeding Your Demons

Anger can become a shadow energy. There is a healthy function for anger, but it needs to be used sparingly and only when appropriate. It would be unwise to assume that there is no place for anger in a spiritual life. The Dalai Lama is very up-front about his anger when others are harmed. Anger is not always putting up walls. It may be necessary to experience our anger in order to go deep and find the source of it.

The non-violent communication (NVC) approach to anger was developed by Marshall Rosenberg. The purpose is to engage in conversation that allows one to find out what is underneath the anger. Often it is pain. The person who wants to fight actually wants to cry. You have to identify in the communication what the person needs in order to heal and how to give that to him or her.

Feeding Your Demons was popularized by Tsultrim Allione. It is a guided visualization for turning emotions like anger, fear, grief, or self-doubt (a demon) into unconditional love, acceptance, or bravery (the ally). This is a very powerful exercise, but it takes time.

The practitioner sits on a blanket or mat with a pillow in front of him or her.

Step 1: Finding the Demon

The guide asks the practitioner, "What is draining your energy? What is causing you pain or anger? Where do you hold this demon in your body? Now observe the demon. What does the demon look like? What color is it? What does it smell like?"

Step 2: Asking the Demon What It Wants of You

The guide tells the practitioner to ask the demon three questions: "What do you want from me? What do you need from me? When this need is met, how will you feel?" The practitioner should take the time he or she needs to ask these questions.

Step 3: Personify the Demon

The practitioner now moves to the pillow and faces where he or she just sat. The practitioner imagines that he or she is the demon responding. The demon says, "What I want from you is. . . . What I need from you is. . . . When my need is met, I will feel. . . ." The practitioner should take the time to feel comfortable becoming the demon and answering the three questions as if he or she were the demon.

Step 4: Feed the Demon

The practitioner moves back to his or her original seat. The guide instructs the practitioner to take what the demon said it needs and imagine this melting into streams of nectar. The practitioner then feeds the nectar to the demon until it is full.

Step 5: Meet the Ally

Imagine the demon taking in the nectar and dissolving into a new being, your ally. What does the ally look like? The practitioner asks the ally four questions: "How will you help me? How will you protect me? What will you pledge to me? How can I gain access to you?"

Step 6: Become the Ally

The practitioner again moves to the pillow. He or she now becomes the ally and answers the four questions that the practitioner asked him or her: "I will help you by. . . . I will protect you by. . . . I will pledge to you. . . . You can gain access to me by. . . ."

Step 7: Relax in Awareness

The practitioner again returns to his or her original seat. He or she imagines the "gifts" that the ally has pledged flowing into nectar that now feeds him or her. The practitioner feels him- or herself integrating into the ally. The practitioner now relaxes in a state of open awareness. This is a natural spaciousness that comes from the dissolution of the demon and the integration into the ally.

[This version of the practice has been modified from the original five steps into seven steps.]

This exercise allows the person to take a difficult emotion like self-doubt and turn it into an ally such as love or grace. The ally could also be a loving friend or family member. The practitioner also learns how he or she can access that feeling of love or grace at any time when he or she feels the demon of self-doubt.[4]

APPENDIX C

Dialogue: When You and Your Spouse Cannot Resolve Conflict

Menopause is a time when women may become more aware of the need to examine unresolved conflicts from their past or may become aware of the need to make changes in their current relationships. Below is the background information and description of a "therapy" that couples can use at home to discuss volatile topics. This information is based on a three-day workshop with psychoanalyst Dr. Polly Young-Eisendarth.[1]

BACKGROUND

We can meet a stranger and develop affection for him or her. Why then do we have so much trouble with those we love?

The universal human self is the experience of being an individual human subject who is:

1. Embodied: We think of our "self" as being inside our body.
2. Continuous: We think of who we are as a continuous narrative/life story/identity. This is a fiction, though. We become a different person about every seven years.
3. Agentive or autonomous: We think there is personal causation associated with our actions. That is, we believe that we are responsible for our own actions.

4. Relational: Our self arises from relating to others. Our self is not inside of us or outside of us but rather the result of relating to other human beings.

We reconstruct events that happened in the past, but we are not very good record keepers. Facts are always interpretive and conditional. We cannot be sure that we are right about the things that have happened. However, we have built our sense of self on this interpretation.

The human self is relational. There is no such thing as a self without other selves. We need others to see and know ourselves. The self becomes solidified from the story line that we tell.

Can the self evolve then without creating "others" outside of the body? We cannot belong without creating others who are against us or our enemies.

There is a certain point in human development (eighteen months to three years old) at which people become protective of who they are. They see that they are separate from the world and inside their body. Children become self-conscious at this point. "I" am "in here," and "you" are "out there."

The archetype of self is activated between infancy and twenty-five years of age. People want to identify with the virtuous; they believe that they know the right way to be. People believe that the "bad" is coming from outside of themselves. It creates feelings of superiority.

Self-consciousness activates the ego or who/what you consider yourself to be.

The mature ego complex or self-consciousness (by the age of twenty-five):

1. I am this kind of person with this identity (narrative/life story).

2. I have this body and identify with being inside it (coherence).

3. I am responsible for or cause my actions and speech (agency/autonomy).

4. I relate to others in my own ways "because of who I am." Through my self-consciousness, I defend my narrative, my coherence, and my agency.

Dependent arising: The "self" and "other" arise together. We need the "other" in order to create the "self."

Psychoanalytic perspective: We are individually motivated to identify with "the good" and either project or ignore "the bad" within our own personalities.

Eventually our partner will disappoint us, and we are set up to make him/ her into "the enemy" or "the other." This is because we put our partners/ lovers on a pedestal early on in the relationship. If we practice love, though, or if it is an intention to abide through all conditions, we can intervene in enemy-making. It is the quality of the attention that we bring to someone we love that prevents us from enemy-making.

Shadow Complex

According to Carl Jung, the primary defense of our own goodness and worth is projection, a move to locate the good or virtuous "in here" while the bad or destructive is "out there." We project the bad or destructive onto others who arise with us in the creation of self. That bad or destructive material comes from the negative parts of our personality, the projection of ourselves as superior or the one who is "right." It also comes from the projection of who we think the other is relative to ourselves or faulty memories of our prior interactions with the other person. Human beings need enemies to manage selves. Homo sapiens are the most violent species and are also very protective and tribal. This can lead to war.

The human condition includes the tendency to create a self, an identity. That self arises simultaneously with the creation of others. We also idealize our partners/lovers. We split off the bad parts of ourselves and project them outside of the group. That is the shadow. We project it onto our partners/lovers when we realize that they are not the ideal people we thought they were. Somebody has to be the scapegoat if there is going to be an ideal. We do not embrace enough within us that is evil. We need to realize that there is negative within us and not project it outward. Evil runs through everyone's heart. The only way to liberate ourselves is to recognize that there is no difference between the self and the other. They arise together.

Mindfulness is the best way to end the cycle of "otherness" leading to hatred and war.

Our most useful enemies are close at hand because we can attempt to control them. We often find them among the people we are supposed to love: our partners, parents, children, lovers, and so on.

The stronger our ideals, the more likely we are to hate those who seem to wreck them. For example, the ideals of equality and reciprocity are especially hard because they invite natural splits and competition of self/ other. The "subject" who projects the harmful "otherness" is dependent on the "object" of that perception because it is the other who defensively defines the self.

From infancy through adulthood, there is a confusing and pervasive emotional communication between people that takes place in a way that reinforces the splits and anxieties about who is doing what to whom. In other words, the projection of "otherness" is confirmed by what the other person does or says, or at least what we think he or she does or says. The receiver of the projection seems to identify with the projected meaning in a way that confirms the projection. This is why people get into repetitive conflicts. We frequently use the people who we are closest to in order to deposit our shadow projections. A couple will need to see each other as separate and different subjectivities in a way that will lead to "no blame" and no need for an enemy.

The Buddha teaches that we are our actions (in speech and deed). Know yourself and others through your actions instead of (1) your embodiment, (2) your narratives, and (3) your relational tribes. Remember: (1) Only 5 percent of your goal-directed actions are conscious, and (2) only 5 percent of the other person's goal-directed actions are conscious.

HOW TO CREATE A MINDFUL SPACE IN RELATION TO THOSE WHO ARISE WITH YOU

1. Recognize yourself as a human being who naturally creates enemies.
2. Reflect on your tendencies and mental habits with the others around you so that you can see why and how you create enemies.
3. Remember that you can cultivate your in-born compassion about your human condition: that you cannot see your disavowed motives clearly and you need others to help you.

Assume:

1. You are aggressive and self-protective; you have a limbic system and an ego complex.
2. You will want to find an enemy in someone in order to protect yourself. Generally, you want this enemy to be close at hand, to be someone who is "supposed to know" what you want and who you are.
3. Be curious about what you are doing when you want to blame another or feel "superior" to someone.

To Love Others or the Self

Become a witness. A witness is someone who sees who we are and who accepts us as we are. We all want to be witnessed. Hold your beloved in mind and remain interested and engaged in him or her through the changes of impermanence. This is true love.

Witnessing depends on:

- Mindfulness, empathy, equanimity, emotional maturity, open communication, and truth-telling
- Willingness and ability to tolerate your own feelings and emotions before acting or speaking

Compassion for the human self is interdependent and unconscious. In order to act consciously, we depend on unconscious processes like projection. We are never completely conscious. Loving ourselves and others cannot be perfected, but it can be embraced as imperfect.

When your limbic system is activated, and you feel emotionally threatened because someone you love has hurt, harmed, or rejected you, connect with your equanimity, your concentration, and your perceptual clarity, and inquire into the dependent arising of self/other.

Dialogue and Witnessing as Antidotes to Projection

Dialogue is a useful skill when you wish to address unresolved conflict with someone you love. It should be used in situations where two people cannot discuss a topic using conventional means. One or both individuals may be aggressive, overreactive, or withdrawn.[2]

The goals of dialogue are to (1) understand the other person's perspective or experience and (2) become a mindful witness to your beloved. We make assumptions about past behaviors and events based on what are often erroneous memories or interpretations. We also project attributes and motivations to the other person in the form of shadow projections. Dialogue allows each individual to clarify those misunderstandings. This requires retaining an open attitude toward your partner, referred to as equanimity. The second goal is to become a mindful witness for your beloved, which includes knowing him or her and accepting him or her deeply. True love is the ability to see your partner clearly and embrace that person as he or she is.[3] In order to see the other person, though, there has to be a space between you. This space is what Young-Eisendrath refers to as a "mindful gap." This means "taking a step back and remembering that you do not know or see or feel exactly or precisely what is going on with your partner or even what is going on with yourself. . . . The first step in becoming a witness [to your beloved] is to . . . never assume you already know."[4]

Prior to dialogue, both parties need to have worked through their own feelings so that they can accurately express them and be aware of their own motivations and desires.

The practice of dialogue works thus:

1. The two individuals sit across from one another. One person starts the dialogue, usually the person who has the concern. That person should explain what he or she sees as the problem, keeping the following in mind:

   a. Speak only for yourself. Use "I" statements instead of "we" statements. Connect to your own subjectivity, feel your feelings, and know what is going on within you.

   b. You should not assume how the other person feels. In fact, one of the goals of the process is to *learn* how the other person does feel or to learn his or her perspective. It is quite likely that either or both persons will learn that their assumptions were not true.

   c. Do not attack or threaten the other person. That will only make him or her defensive and angry. Be kind and authentic. Do not use statements such as "You did this . . ." or "You never. . . ." Avoid statements like "I feel really upset when you cut off the conversation." Instead, say, "I feel very upset when I feel overlooked or cut off."

   d. Be clear and empathic. Remember that you are trying to understand how the other person sees things as well as to convey your own perspective. Try putting yourself in the other person's shoes. Likewise, be as clear as possible so that the other person can understand your perspective.

   e. Cultivate equanimity. Equanimity is a calm, centered acceptance of your own feelings and internal agitation.

   f. Be an active and deep listener. Speak and listen with an open heart.

2. The other person will then *paraphrase* what the first person said, using the same five principles explained above. Young-Eisendrath writes:

Paraphrasing is the act of stepping back from your own defensiveness and reactivity. It opens the space to a mindful gap in which you can both feel your own feelings and concentrate on your partner's words and feelings. True paraphrasing, like true empathy, means that you try to step into your partner's experience and infer what it's like for your partner."[5]

3. After paraphrasing, the person will ask his or her partner if he or she has summarized the other person's feelings accurately. If the partner says no, then the person should ask the partner what he or she has misunderstood. Then the participant will paraphrase again and ask if this is correct. The process should continue back and forth like this until the second person has paraphrased the first person's concerns accurately.

4. After correctly paraphrasing the first person's concerns, the second person has an opportunity to respond. He or she may ask questions of the first person, such as asking him or her to clarify. The second person may also choose to explain his or her own perspective or to clarify how his or her intentions were different from what was assumed.

5. Now the first person paraphrases what the partner said and asks if he or she has summarized their perspective accurately. Again, they go back and forth until they arrive at a correct paraphrasing.

6. The partners will continue to explain their perspectives and interpretations until each clearly understands the other person's position. Each should also ask (in turn) if there is something that the other person would like to add. It is quite likely that one or both individuals will apologize during the process.

7. The partners should be curious and ask questions to better understand their beloved. They will continue going back and forth, paraphrasing and asking questions until they come to a solution or resolution that seems to work for both of them. Through dialogue, partners will become more empathic and sympathetic of the other person.

8. If the process does not seem to work, the couple may need initial assistance from a skilled psychoanalyst(s). Psychoanalysts who work with couples often work in pairs. Each analyst will serve as one of the partner's coach and/or alter ego and assist them in learning to express themselves and recognize their own motivations and desires.

In time the couple will be skilled in equanimity and in concentrating on what each partner is saying in a discussion. They will no longer need a formal dialogue session but can instead rely on regular discussion. Each person will be able to see him- or herself through a new lens and begin to understand how his or her own history and earlier relationships may make current struggles so painful and/or lead to shadow projections. He or she will begin to understand what is happening when triggered by unconscious themes that the partner is actually not responsible for.

The goal of meditation and exercises like the one above is to create a space for people to think about how they wish to respond rather than reacting automatically. We have the freedom to step back and respond in a way that does not perpetuate misunderstandings or old family patterns. It also increases the likelihood of letting an experience move through us rather than clinging to it or to the story line that we have assigned to it. We recognize that the assumptions that we have considered facts may not be true and that we have projected our own negativity onto the other person. We recognize that other people are also under conditions and circumstances that have caused them to act the way that they do.

Before saying something to someone else, first T.H.I.N.K. Make sure that what you are about to say passes the test of being kind, true, and necessary.

T: Is what you have to say TRUE and not an assumption or your own perspective?

N: Is what you have to say NECESSARY? Will it benefit the other person or you?

K: Is what you have to say KIND? If not, can you find a kind way to say it?

The following meditation helps to anchor an individual to the present moment. It is a shikantaza meditation, translated to mean "sitting like a rock." By "sitting like a rock," the practitioner does not get pulled and pushed by that which surrounds him or her. This meditation will also show you just how much of what you are experiencing comes from you and is not objective fact. Remembering that will allow you to work with your subjective experience without reacting to or blowing up at the other person. The meditation is described in the following section.

Opening Our Sense Gates Meditation

1. Sit in a comfortable position with a straight back, hands loose on your lap.

2. Hear "in": Say to yourself, "Hear in," and hear the voices in your head. What are you saying to yourself? Hear your own heartbeat, your own breath. Hear the sounds inside of your body for two to three minutes.

3. Hear "out": Now listen for any sounds outside of your body. Say to yourself, "Hear out." What sounds in your environment can you hear? Is there a clock ticking? Do you hear traffic off in the distance? Are there people talking? What sounds in the environment can you hear?

4. See "in": Say to yourself, "See in." What do you see in your mind's eye? What are the colors? You might want to imagine a scene. What are the details of that scene? Spend two to three minutes on what you see.

5. See "out": Now open your eyes. Without moving your head, look to see what is within your range of sight. Say to yourself, "See out."

6. Feel "in": Close your eyes once again. Feel in to your emotional centers, the chakras. What emotions are you feeling? Say to yourself, "Feel in."

7. Feel "out": Feel the body as it is presenting itself. Can you feel your clothing on your skin? Is the wind blowing on your face? Can you feel the pressure of your sit bones on your chair? Notice what you feel from outside of your body for two to three minutes.

With practice, you will eventually be able to ground yourself at any time during the day by saying "Hear in" (or any of the other prompts) and bring yourself back to the present moment.

APPENDIX D

Resources for Meditation and Mindfulness

BOOKS ABOUT MINDFULNESS AND MEDITATION

Begley, Sharon. *Train Your Mind, Change Your Brain.* New York: Ballantine Books, 2007.

Brach, Tara. *True Refuge: Finding Peace and Freedom in Your Own Awakened Heart.* New York: Bantam Books, 2013.

Cayton, Karuna. *The Misleading Mind: How We Create Our Own Problems and How Buddhist Psychology Can Help Us Solve Them.* Novato, CA: New World Library, 2012.

Chödrön, Pema. *Living Beautifully with Uncertainty and Change.* Boston, MA: Shambhala, 2012.

Chödrön, Pema. *The Places That Scare You: A Guide to Fearlessness in Difficult Times.* Boulder, CO: Shambhala Classics, 2002.

Davidson, Richard J. with Sharon Begley. *The Emotional Life of Your Brain.* New York: Plume, 2013.

Germer, Christopher K. *The Mindful Path to Self-Compassion.* New York: The Guilford Press, 2009.

Hanh, Thich Nhat. *Peace Is Every Step: The Path of Mindfulness in Everyday Life.* New York: Bantam Books, 1991.

Moffitt, Phillip. *Dancing with Life: Buddhist Insights for Finding Meaning and Joy in the Face of Suffering.* New York: Rodale Inc., 2008.

Neff, Kristen. *Self-Compassion: The Proven Power of Being Kind to Yourself.* New York: Harper Collins Publishers, 2011.

Piver, Susan. *Start Here Now: An Open-Hearted Guide to the Path and Practice of Meditation.* Boston, MA: Shambhala, 2015.

Siegel, Daniel J. *Mindsight: The New Science of Personal Transformation.* New York: Bantam Books, 2010.

Williams, Mark, John Teasdale, Zindel Segal, and Jon Kabat-Zinn. *The Mindful Way through Depression.* New York: The Guilford Press, 2007.

MEDITATION AND SELF-COMPASSION VIDEOS

Brach, Tara: https://www.tarabrach.com/practical-dharma-for-stressful-times-audio

Chödrön, Pema: https://www.lionsroar.com/pema-chodron

Neff, Kristen: https://www.youtube.com/watch?v=rUMF5R7DoOA

FREE APPS

https://buddhify.com
https://insighttimer.com
https://wa-health-Kaiserpermanente.org/best-meditation-apps/
https://www.headspace.com
https://www.mindful.org/free-mindfulness-apps-worthy-of-your-attention/
https://www.self.com/gallery/free-meditation-apps

COURSES IN MINDFULNESS AND MEDITATION

Engaged Mindfulness Institute: engagedmindfulness.org

Inward Bound Mindfulness Education (throughout the United States): https://ibme.com. (978) 254-7082

Mindfulness Differently (Berkeley, CA, and online): www.fullpresence.org

University of Massachusetts Medical School (Worcester, MA): https://www.umassmed.edu/cfm

- Mindfulness-Based Stress Reduction (MBSR) program
- Mindfulness-Based Cognitive Therapy (MBCT) program

YOGA

www.YogisOnTheGo.com

Notes

CHAPTER 1

1. Centre for Menstrual Cycle and Ovulation Research, 2018, www .cmcor.ubc.ca/resources.

2. Mayo Clinic, 2018, https://www.mayoclinic.org/diseases-conditions /menopause.

3. Boston Women's Health Book Collective, *Our Bodies, Ourselves: Menopause* (New York: Simon and Schuster, 2006), 4.

4. Ibid.

5. Mayo Clinic.

6. Centre for Menstrual Cycle and Ovulation Research.

7. Boston Women's Health Book Collective, *Our Bodies, Ourselves.*

8. Centre for Menstrual Cycle and Ovulation Research.

9. Amy Hendel, reviewed by Peter J. Chen, M.D., FACOG, "Ten Things You Should Know About Menopause," HealthCentral.com (November 2, 2012).

10. Pat Wingert and Barbara Kantrowitz, *The Menopause Book*, 2nd ed. (New York: Workman Publishing, 2009).

11. Hot flashes refer to episodes of feeling extremely hot to the point of discomfort. Many women said that they would sweat during a hot flash and wished that they could take their clothes off during these episodes. For some women, the hot flash would begin in their toes and travel to their heads. Hot flashes could occur at any time of the day. Elyse said that she experienced as many as twenty hot flashes per day before seeking HRT. Hot flashes could last five to fifteen minutes.

12. Vaginal dryness that results in painful intercourse is referred to as dyspareunia in the medical community.

13. Night sweats occur exclusively while sleeping. They result from hot flashes causing women to wake up "drenched in sweat" and needing to change their bed clothes. Most of the women who had night sweats had one or two per night, but some had as few as one every three or four days. Night sweats exacerbated insomnia because the women needed to fall back to sleep after waking and/or changing their clothing.

14. Bindhu S. Anil, Bhaskar Anitha, and Joseph Jose, "Prevalence of Menopausal Symptoms among Women (Menopausal for <5 Years) in a Rural Area in Kottayam, Kerala, India," *Journal of Evolution of Medical and Dental Sciences* 3, no. 17 (April 28, 2014): 4648–60.

15. Jane E. Brody, "The Stubborn Markers of Menopause," *New York Times* (February 11, 2014): Section D, 5.

16. Christiane Northrup, MD, *The Wisdom of Menopause* (New York: Bantam Books, 2012).

17. Kari Oakes, "Chronic Insomnia Affects One-Third in Menopause," *Clinical Psychiatry News* 44, no. 1 (January, 2016): 27.

18. Writing Group for the Women's Health Initiative Investigation, "Risk and Benefits of Estrogen and Progestin in Healthy Postmenopausal Women," *Journal of the American Medical Association* 268 (2002): 321–33.

19. Shumin M. Zhang, JoAnn E. Manson, Kathryn M. Rexrode, Nancy R. Cook, Julie E. Burning, and I-Min Lee, "Use of Oral Conjugated Estrogen Alone and Risk of Breast Cancer," *American Journal of Epidemiology* 165, no. 5 (March 1, 2007): 524–29.

20. Brody, "Stubborn Markers of Menopause."

21. Northrup, *Wisdom of Menopause.*

22. Hendel, "Ten Things You Should Know About Menopause."

23. Centers for Disease Control, "Leading Cause of Death in Females, United States," 2015, https://www.cdc.gov/women/lcod/index.htm.

24. Mia Lundin, *Female Brain Gone Insane* (Deerfield Beach, FL: Health Communications Inc., 2009).

25. Andrea Chisholm, MD, "Menopause Treatments," October 18, 2016, http://www.verywellhealth.menopause.about.com.treatment.

26. Ibid.

27. Sara Gottfried, MD, and Christiane Northrup, MD, *The Hormone Cure: Reclaim Balance, Sleep, and Sex Drive—Lose Weight, Feel Focused, Vital and Energized Naturally with the Gottfried Protocol* (New York: Scribner, 2014).

28. John R. Lee and Virginia Hopkins, *What Your Doctor May Not Tell You about Menopause: The Breakthrough Book on Natural Hormone Balance* (New York: Warner Books, 2004).

29. Jenna Fletcher, "Bioidentical Hormones: How Are They Used?" *Medical News Today* (September 19, 2017), http://medicalnewstoday.com/articles/319465.php.

30. Chisholm, "Menopause Treatments."

31. Paige Waehner, "Ease into Menopause with Exercise," 2016, http://www.verywell.com/ease-into-menopause-with-exercise-1231560.

32. Melinda Ring, *The Natural Menopause Solution: Expert Advice for Melting Stubborn Midlife Pounds, Reducing Hot Flashes, and Getting Relief from Menopause Symptoms* (New York: Rodale Books, 2012).

33. Waehner, "Ease into Menopause with Exercise."

34. Chisholm, "Menopause Treatments."

35. Hendel, "Ten Things You Should Know about Menopause."

36. *Herbalist Report*, "Menopause Support Report 2017," 2017, www.herbalistreport.com/menopause-herbal-solutions-bing/index2.html.

37. Ring, *Natural Menopause Solution*.

38. S. Basaria et al., "Effect of High-Dose Isoflavones on Cognition, Quality of Life, Androgens, and Lipoprotein in Post-Menopausal Women," *Journal of Endocrinological Investigation* 32, no. 2 (2009): 150–55.

39. Lundin, *Female Brain Gone Insane*.

40. Carolyn Ambler Walter, "The Psychosocial Meaning of Menopause: Women's Experiences," *Journal of Women and Aging* 12, no. 3/4 (2000): 117–31.

41. Ibid., p. 120.

42. Ibid.

43. Gail Sheehy, *Passages: Predictable Crises of Adult Life* (New York: Ballantine Books, 2006).

44. Gail Sheehy, *The Silent Passage: Menopause* (New York: Pocket Books, 2010).

45. Carolyn Ambler Walter, "The Psychosocial Meaning of Menopause: Women's Experiences," *Journal of Women and Aging* 12, no. 3/4 (2000): 122.

46. Northrup, *Wisdom of Menopause*.

47. Walter, "Psychosocial Meaning."

48. Northrup, *Wisdom of Menopause*, p. 9.

49. Ibid., p. 19.

50. Lundin, *Female Brain Gone Insane*.

51. Northrup, *Wisdom of Menopause*, p. 65.

52. Robert A. Wilson and Thelma A. Wilson, "The Fate of the Non-treated Postmenopausal Woman: A Plea for the Maintenance of Adequate Estrogen from Puberty to the Grave," *Journal of the American Geriatrics Society* 11 (1963): 347–62.

53. Office for National Statistics, "How Has Life Expectancy Changed over Time?" September 9, 2015, http://www.visual.ons.gov.uk/how-has -life-expectancy-changed-over-time.

CHAPTER 2

1. Betty Friedan, *The Fountain of Age* (New York: Simon and Schuster, 1993).

2. Ibid., p. 44.

3. Gail Sheehy, *The Silent Passage: Menopause* (New York: Pocket Books, 2010).

4. https://www.imdb.com/title/tt0509864.

5. https://www.imdb.com/title/tt0589742.

6. The author attended *Menopause The Musical* in April 2016.

7. The magazines included *Woman's Day, Good Housekeeping, Southern Lady, Moves: Lifestyle for City Women, Women's Health, Dr. Oz: The Good Life*, and *O, The Oprah Magazine*. These were selected as magazines that would appeal to women of myriad interests. Magazines from November 2017 to November 2018 were analyzed.

8. www.menopause.org. Accessed December 6, 2018.

9. https://redhotmamas.org. Accessed December 6, 2018.

10. https://menopausegoddessblog.com. Accessed December 6, 2018.

11. https://ellendolgen.com. Accessed December 6, 2018.

12. Judith A. Houck, *Hot and Bothered: Medicine and Menopause in Modern America* (Cambridge, MA: Harvard University Press, 2006).

13. Office for National Statistics, "How Has Life Expectancy Changed Over Time?" September 9, 2015, http://www.visual.ons.gov.uk/how-has -life-expectancy-changed-over-time.

14. Thomas Bodenheimer and Kevin Grumbach, "Paying for Health Care," in *The Sociology of Health and Illness* (New York: Worth Publishers, 2013), 326–36.

15. Peter Conrad and Valerie Leiter, "From Lydia Pinkham to Queen Levitra: Direct-to-Consumer Advertising and Medicalization," in *The Sociology of Health and Illness*, Peter Conrad and Valerie Leiter, eds. (New York: Worth Publishers, 2013), 301–11.

16. Houck, *Hot and Bothered*.

17. Ibid.

18. Robert A. Wilson and Thelma A. Wilson, "The Fate of the Non-treated Postmenopausal Woman: A Plea for the Maintenance of Adequate

Estrogen from Puberty to the Grave," *Journal of the American Geriatrics Society* 11 (1963): 347–62.

19. David Reuben, *Everything You Wanted to Know about Sex: But Were Afraid to Ask* (New York: David McKay Co., 1969), 290.

20. Newsweek Staff, "No More Menopause," *Newsweek* (January 13, 1964): 53.

21. Vogue Staff, "How to Live Young at Any Age," *Vogue* (August 1965): 61–64.

22. Sherwin A. Kaufman, "The Truth about Female Hormones," *Ladies Home Journal* (January 1965): 22–23.

23. Cosmopolitan Staff, "Oh What a Lovely Pill," *Cosmopolitan* (July 1965): 33–37.

24. Robert A. Wilson and Thelma A. Wilson, *Feminine Forever* (New York: M. Evans and Company, 1966).

25. Ann Walsh, *E.R.T.: The Pills to Keep Women Young* (New York: Bantam, 1965).

26. Houck, *Hot and Bothered.*

27. Writing Group for the Women's Health Initiative Investigation, "Risk and Benefits of Estrogen and Progestin in Healthy Postmenopausal Women," *Journal of the American Medical Association* 268 (2002): 321–33.

28. Vicki Hart, Susan R. Sturgeon, Nicholas Reich, Lynette Leidy Sievert, Sibyl L. Crawford, and Ellen B. Gold, "Menopausal Vasomotor Symptoms and Incident Breast Cancer Risk in the Study of Women's Health Across the Nation," *Cancer Causes and Control* 27, no. 11 (November 2016): 1333.

29. Andrea Chisholm, MD, "Menopause Treatments," October 18, 2016, http://www.verywellhealth.menopause.about.treatment.com.

30. Mia Lundin, *Female Brain Gone Insane* (Deerfield Beach, FL: Health Communications Inc., 2009).

31. Chisholm, "Menopause Treatments."

32. Harvard Health Letter, April 30, 2018, www.health.harvard.edu/mind-and-mood/exercise-is-an-all-natural-treatment-to-fight-depression.

33. Chisholm, "Menopause Treatments."

34. Amy Hendel, "Ten Things You Should Know about Menopause," HealthCentral.com, November 2, 2012.

35. Herbalist Report, "Menopause Support Report 2017," 2017, www.herbalistreport.com/menopause-herbal-solutions-bing/index2.html.

36. Melinda Ring, *The Natural Menopause Solution: Expert Advice for Melting Stubborn Midlife Pounds, Reducing Hot Flashes, and Getting Relief from Menopause Symptoms* (New York: Rodale Books, 2012).

37. Christiane Northrup, MD, "Do You Need Bioidentical Hormones?" September 11, 2017, https://www.drnorthrup.com/do-you-need-bioidentical-hormones.

38. Christiane Northrup, MD, "Herbs to Relieve Menopause Symptoms," September 11, 2017, https://www.drnorthrup.com/traditional-herbs-or-bioidentical-hormones-which-is-better.

39. S. Basaria et al., "Effect of High-Dose Isoflavones on Cognition, Quality of Life, Androgens, and Lipoprotein in Post-Menopausal Women," *Journal of Endocrinological Investigation* 32, no. 2 (2009): 150–55.

40. Mindfulness specifically refers to being aware of one's thoughts, emotions, and bodily sensations as they occur. On a higher level, it refers to being aware of what is happening in the present without wishing that it were different, enjoying the pleasant without holding on when it changes, and being with the unpleasant without fear that it will always remain. It is a process of recognizing one's thoughts and emotions and allowing them to flow through the mind and body without hanging on to them. See James Baraz and Shoshana Alexander, *Awakening Joy* (Berkeley, CA: Parallax Press, 2012).

41. James Francis Carmody, Sybil Crawford, Elena Salmoirago-Blotcher, Katherine Leung, Linda Churchill, and Nicholas Olendzki, "Mindfulness Training for Coping with Hot Flashes," *Menopause* 18, no. 6 (2011): 611–20.

42. Jeena Cho, "The Science behind How Mindfulness Helps You to Break Negative Thought Patterns," *Forbes Magazine* (December 27, 2016), http://www.forbes.com/sites/jeenacho/2016/12/27/the-science-behind-how-mindfulness-helps-you-to-break-negative-though-patterns/#3a0e0482f83a.

43. Teper Rimma, Zindel V. Segal, and Michael Inzlicht, "Inside the Mindful Mind: How Mindfulness Enhances Emotion Regulation through Improvement in Executive Control," *Current Directions in Psychological Science* 22 (2013): 449–54.

44. Yi-Yuan Tang, Britta K. Holzel, and Michael I. Posner, "The Neuroscience of Mindfulness Meditation," *Nature Reviews Neuroscience* 16 (March 18, 2015): 213–25.

45. Richard J. Davidson, Jon Kabat-Zinn, J. Schumacher, M. Rosenkranz, D. Muller, S. Santorelli, et al., "Alterations in Brain and Immune Function Produced by Mindfulness Meditation," *Psychosomatic Medicine* 65, no. 4 (2003): 564–70.

46. Sara Lazar, C. Kerr, R. Wasserman, J. Gray, D. Greve, M. Treadway, et al., "Meditation Experience Is Associated with Increased Cortical Thickness," *NeuroReport* 16, no. 17 (2005): 1893–97.

47. Christopher K. Germer, *The Mindful Path to Self-Compassion* (New York: The Guilford Press, 2009).

48. E. L. Garland, S. A. Gaylord, and B. L. Frederickson, "Positive Reappraisal Mediates the Stress-Reductive Effects of Mindfulness: An Upward Spiral Process," *Mindfulness* 2 (2011): 59–67.

49. Germer, *Mindful Path to Self-Compassion*.

50. Emily K. Lindsay and J. David Creswell, "Back to Basics: How Attention Monitoring and Acceptance Stimulate Positive Growth," *Psychological Inquiry* 26 (2015): 343–48.

51. Ibid., p. 347.

52. Germer, *Mindful Path to Self-Compassion*, p. 118.

53. Mia Lundin, *Female Brain Gone Insane* (Deerfield Beach, FL: Health Communications Inc., 2009).

54. Boston Women's Health Book Collective, *Our Bodies, Ourselves: Menopause* (New York: Simon and Schuster, 2006).

55. Robert A. Wilson and Thelma A. Wilson, "The Fate of Nontreated Menopausal Woman: A Plea for the Maintenance of Adequate Estrogen from Puberty to the Grave," *Journal of American Geriatrics Society* 11 (1963): 347–62.

56. Houck, *Hot and Bothered*.

57. Chisholm, "Menopause Treatments."

58. Lundin, *Female Brain Gone Insane*.

59. Northrup, *Wisdom of Menopause*, p. 19.

CHAPTER 3

1. Christiane Northrup, MD, *The Wisdom of Menopause* (New York: Bantam Books, 2012).

2. Perimenopause and menopause typically include both symptoms affecting temperament and physical symptoms.

3. Interview with Dr. Victoria Delgado, DO, Reliant Medical Group, St. Vincent Hospital, Worcester, Massachusetts, October 6, 2014.

4. Sharon Begley, *Train Your Mind, Change Your Brain* (New York: Ballantine Books, 2007).

5. James Francis Carmody, Sybil Crawford, Elena Salmoirago-Blotcher, Katherine Leung, Linda Churchill, and Nicholas Olendzki, "Mindfulness Training for Coping with Hot Flashes," *Menopause* 18, no. 6 (2011): 611–20.

6. Daniel J. Siegel, *Mindsight: The New Science of Personal Transformation* (New York: Bantam Books, 2010).

7. Mark Williams, John Teasdale, Zindel Segal, and Jon Kabat-Zinn, *The Mindful Way through Depression* (New York: The Guilford Press, 2007).

8. Carmody et al., "Mindfulness Training."

9. Interview with Dr. Victoria Delgado, DO.

10. Endometriosis is a painful condition where the endometrium, or tissue that lines the uterus, grows outside of the uterus. It may involve the ovaries, fallopian tubes, and/or the pelvis. (Mayo Clinic, July 24, 2018, https://www.mayoclinic.org/diseases-conditions/endometriosis.)

11. The Boston Women's Health Collective, *Our Bodies, Ourselves: Menopause* (New York: Simon and Schuster, 2006).

12. Ibid.

13. Ibid.

CHAPTER 4

1. Sally Dammery, *First Blood: A Cultural Study of Menarche* (Clayton, Victoria, Australia: Monash University Publishing, 2016).

2. Rebecca Utz, "Like Mother, (Not) Like Daughter: The Social Construction of Menopause and Aging," *Journal of Aging Studies* 25 (2011): 143–54.

3. Ibid., p. 143.

4. Ibid., p. 147.

5. Robert A. Wilson and Thelma A. Wilson, *Feminine Forever* (New York: M. Evans Company, 1966).

6. Utz, "Like Mother, (Not) Like Daughter," p. 150.

7. Gail Sheehy, *The Silent Passage: Menopause* (New York: Pocket Books, 2010).

8. Utz, "Like Mother, (Not) Like Daughter," p. 152.

9. Sheehy, *Silent Passage*.

10. Ibid., Pauline Bart, p. 58.

11. Ibid., Bateson, p. 58.

12. Daniel Delanoe, Selma Jajri, Annie Bachelot, Dorra Mahfoudh Draoui, Danielle Hassoun, Elise Marsicano, and Virginie Ringa, "Class, Gender, and Culture in the Experience of Menopause: A Comparative Study in Tunisia and France," *Social Science and Medicine* 75 (2012): 401–9.

13. Sheehy, *Silent Passage*. This refers to a study by Margaret Locke, p. 59.

14. Zhao Feng, "Construction of Menopause: An Inquiry of Cultural Influences on Menopause and Associated Problems" (paper presented at the annual meetings of the American Sociological Association, Atlanta, Georgia, August 16, 2003).

15. Sheehy, *Silent Passage*.

16. Ibid.

17. Julie A. Winterich, "From Biology to Culture: The Roles of Gender, Race, and Sexuality for Women's Menopausal Experiences" (paper presented at the annual meetings of the American Sociological Association, Atlanta, Georgia, August 16, 2003).

18. Heather E. Dillaway, "Why Can't You Control This? How Women's Interactions with Intimate Partners Define Menopause and Family," *Journal of Women and Aging* 20, no. 1 (2008): 47–64.

19. Heather E. Dillaway, "(Un)Changing Menopausal Bodies: How Women Think and Act in the Face of Reproductive Transition and Gendered Body Ideals," *Sex Roles* 53, no. 1/2 (July 2005): 1–17.

20. Ibid.

21. Lynn A. Morrison, Lynnette L. Sievert, Daniel E. Brown, Nichole Rahberg, and Angela Reza, "Relationships between Menstrual and Menopausal Attitudes and Associated Demographic and Health Characteristics: The Hilo Women's Health Study," *Women and Health* 50 (2010): 397–413.

22. Judy R. Strauss, "Contextual Influences on Women's Health Concerns and Attitudes towards Menopause," *Health and Social Work* 36, no. 2 (May 2011): 121–27.

23. Judy R. Strauss, "The Baby Boomers Meet Menopause: Fertility, Attractiveness, and Affective Responses to the Menopausal Transition," *Sex Roles* 68 (2013): 77–90.

24. Michelle R. Newhart, "Menopause Matters: The Implications of Menopause Research for Studies of Midlife Health," *Health Sociology Review* 22, no. 4 (2013): 365–76.

25. Delanoe et al., "Class, Gender, and Culture."

26. Betty Friedan, *The Fountain of Age* (New York: Simon and Schuster, 1993).

27. Robert A. Wilson and Thelma A. Wilson, "The Fate of the Nontreated Postmenopausal Woman: A Plea for the Maintenance of Adequate Estrogen from Puberty to the Grave," *Journal of the American Geriatrics Society* 11 (1963): 347–62.

28. Wilson and Wilson, *Feminine Forever*.

CHAPTER 5

1. Heather E. Dillaway and Mary Byrnes, "Talking 'Among Us': Racial and Ethnic Perspectives of the Menopausal Experience" (paper presented at the annual meetings of the American Sociological Association, Montreal, Canada, August 2006).

2. Sarah Spettel and Mark Donald White, "The Portrayal of J. Marion Sims' Controversial Surgical Legacy," *The Journal of Urology* 185 (June 2011): 2424–27.

3. L. L. Wall, "The Medical Ethics of Dr. J. Marion Sims: A Fresh Look at the Historical Record," *Journal of Medical Ethics* 32, no. 6 (June 2006): 346–50.

4. Sarah Zhang, "The Surgeon Who Experimented on Slaves," *Atlantic* (April 18, 2018).

5. Dillaway and Byrnes, "Talking 'Among Us.'"

6. Ibid.

7. Ibid.

8. Julie A. Winterich and Debra Umberson, "How Women Experience Menopause: The Importance of Social Context," *Journal of Women and Aging* 11, no. 4 (1999): 57–73.

9. Gail Sheehy, *The Silent Passage: Menopause* (New York: Pocket Books, 2010).

10. Ibid.

11. Joyce T. Broomberger, Peter M. Meyer, Howard M. Kravitz, Barbara Sommer, Adriana Cordal, Lynda Powell, Patricia A. Ganz, and Kim Sutton-Tyrell, "Psychologic Distress and Natural Menopause: A Multiethnic Community Study," *American Journal of Public Health* 91, no. 9 (September 2001): 1435–42.

12. Sheehy, *Silent Passage*.

13. Michelle R. Newhart, "Menopause Matters: The Implications of Menopause Research for Studies of Midlife Health," *Health Sociology Review* 22, no. 4 (2013): 365–76.

14. M. Breheny and C. Stephens, "Healthy Living and Keeping Busy: A Discourse Analysis of Mid-Aged Women's Attributions for Menopausal Experience," *Journal of Language and Social Psychology* 22, no. 2 (2003): 169–89.

15. Dillaway and Byrnes, "Talking 'Among Us.'"

16. Endometriosis is a painful disorder that occurs when the tissue that normally lines the inside of the uterus grows on the outside of the

uterus and, potentially, the fallopian tubes, ovaries, and pelvic region. The displaced tissue bleeds and sheds itself during menstruation just like in the uterus, but there is no place for it to go. The tissue becomes irritated, and cysts may develop, typically on the ovaries. It can result in infertility if not corrected. See Boston Women's Health Collective and Judy Norsigian, *Our Bodies, Ourselves* (New York: Simon and Schuster, 2011).

17. Henrietta Lacks, a black woman, was the source of the HeLa cell line. Henrietta had a tumor biopsied during treatment for cervical cancer in 1951. Unbeknown to her, the cells were kept and found to be able to live outside of the body and reproduce infinitely. The cells were then used extensively in medical research. It was not until the 1970s though that her family was told of their mother's role in this research. It is the family's belief that they have not received adequate compensation on their mother's behalf. See Rebecca Skloot, *The Immortal Life of Henrietta Lacks* (New York: Crown Publishing Group, 2010).

18. Dillaway and Byrnes, "Talking 'Among Us.'"

19. Susan Sontag, *Illness as Metaphor and AIDS and Its Metaphors* (New York: Picador, 2001).

CHAPTER 6

1. Christiane Northrup, MD, *The Wisdom of Menopause* (New York: Bantam Books, 2012), 19.

2. Ibid.

3. Simon B. Goldberg, Raymond P. Tucker, Preston A. Greene, David J. Kearney, and Tracy L. Simpson, "Mindfulness-Based Interventions for Psychiatric Disorders: A Systematic Review and Meta-analysis," *Clinical Psychology Review* 59 (February 2018): 52–60.

4. Mark Williams, John Teasdale, Zindel Segal, and Jon Kabat-Zinn, *The Mindful Way through Depression* (New York: The Guilford Press, 2007).

5. Mindful Staff, "Jon Kabat-Zinn: Defining Mindfulness," January 11, 2017, www.mindful.org.

6. Ryan M. Niemiec, "3 Definitions of Mindfulness That Might Surprise You," *Psychology Today* (November 1, 2017), https://www.psychologytoday.com.

7. Tara Brach, *True Refuge* (New York: Bantam Books, 2013).

8. Ruminating refers to focusing on the same thoughts over and over again.

9. Jeena Cho, "The Science Behind How Mindfulness Helps You to Break Negative Thought Patterns," *Forbes Magazine* (December 27, 2016).

10. Emily K. Lindsay and J. David Creswell, "Back to Basics: How Attention Monitoring and Acceptance Stimulate Positive Growth," *Psychological Inquiry* 26 (2015): 343–48.

11. Teper Rimma, Zindel V. Segal, and Michael Inzlicht, "Inside the Mindful Mind: How Mindfulness Enhances Emotion Regulation Through Improvements in Executive Control," *Current Directions in Psychological Science* 22 (2013): 449–54.

12. James Baraz and Shoshana Alexander, *Awakening Joy* (Berkeley, CA: Parallax Press, 2012).

13. Sharon Begley, *Train Your Mind, Change Your Brain* (New York: Ballantine Books, 2007).

14. Richard J. Davidson with Sharon Begley, *The Emotional Life of Your Brain* (New York: Plume, 2013).

15. Daniel J. Siegel, *Mindsight: The New Science of Personal Transformation* (New York: Bantam Books, 2010).

16. Yi-Yuan Tang, Britta K. Holzel, and Michael I. Posner, "The Neuroscience of Mindfulness Meditation," *Nature Reviews Neuroscience* 16 (March 18, 2015): 213–25.

17. Baraz and Alexander, *Awakening Joy.*

18. James Francis Carmody, Sybil Crawford, Elena Salmoirago-Blotcher, Katherine Leung, Linda Churchill, and Nicholas Olendzki, "Mindfulness Training for Coping with Hot Flashes," *Menopause* 18, no. 6 (2011): 611–20.

19. Northrup, *Wisdom of Menopause*, p. 37.

20. Northrup, *Wisdom of Menopause.*

21. Ibid.

22. Ibid., p. 58.

23. Nina's first husband was killed in a bicycling accident.

24. Cynthia later learned that only one provider in her area accepted her insurance unconditionally, whereas other providers took only one patient with her insurance at a time due to the insurance company's low reimbursement.

25. Cynthia later learned that she could see the nurse practitioner only if she was seeing a therapist and vice versa.

26. Northrup, *Wisdom of Menopause*, p. 19.

CHAPTER 7

1. Sharon E. Robinson Kurpius, Megan Foley Nicpon, and Susan E. Maresh, "Mood, Marriage, and Menopause," *Journal of Counseling Psychology* 48, no. 1 (2001): 77–84.

2. Katherine Vaughn Fielder and Sharon E. Robinson Kurpius, "Marriage, Stress, and Menopause: Midlife Challenges and Joys," *Psicologia* 19, no. 1–2 (2005): 87–106.

3. Steriani Elavsly and Edward McAuley, "Physical Activity, Symptoms, Esteem, and Life Satisfaction during Menopause," *Maturitas* 52, no. 3–4 (2005): 374–85.

4. Fielder and Kurpius, "Marriage, Stress, and Menopause."

5. For example, one of the women had lost her husband to cancer in the past year. Although she was still grieving the loss, she said that she was grateful that he was no longer suffering.

6. Harry R. Moody and Jennifer R. Sasser, *Aging Concepts and Controversies* (Los Angeles, CA: Sage Publications, 2015).

7. Ibid.

8. Christiane Northrup, *The Wisdom of Menopause* (New York: Bantam Books, 2012), 319–20.

9. Ibid., p. 319.

10. Heather E. Dillaway, "Menopause Is the 'Good Old': Women's Thoughts about Reproductive Aging," *Gender and Society* 19, no. 3 (June 2005): 398–417.

11. L. A. Gavrilov and N. S. Gravrilova, "New Findings on Human Longevity Predictors" (paper presented at the annual meeting of the Gerontological Society of America, San Francisco, California, November 19, 2007).

12. S. T. Lindau et al., "A Study of the Sexuality and Health among Older Adults in the United States," *New England Journal of Medicine* 357 (2007): 762–74.

13. U. Hartmann et al., "Low Sexual Desire in Midlife and Older Women: Personality Factors, Psychosocial Development, Present Sexuality," *Menopause* 11, no. 6 (2004): 726–40.

14. Northrup, *The Wisdom of Menopause.*

15. D. Wilson, "Drug for Sexual Disorder Opposed by Panel," *New York Times* B3, June 19, 2010, www.nytimes.com/2010/06/19/business/19 sexpill.html.

16. Northrup, *Wisdom of Menopause*, p. 325.

CHAPTER 8

1. Daniel Siegel, *Aware: The Science and Practice of Presence* (New York: TarcherPerigee, 2018).

2. Susan Piver, *Start Here Now: An Open-Hearted Guide to the Path and Practice of Meditation* (Boston, MA: Shambhala Publications, 2015).

3. Pema Chödrön, *The Places That Scare You: A Guide to Fearlessness in Difficult Times* (Boulder, CO: Shambhala Publications, 2002).

4. Thich Nhat Hahn, *The Heart of the Buddha's Teaching: Transforming Suffering into Peace, Joy, and Liberation* (New York: Harmony Books, 2015).

5. Tara Brach, *True Refuge: Finding Peace and Freedom in Your Own Awakened Heart* (New York: Bantam Books, 2013).

6. Pema Chödrön, *Living Beautifully with Uncertainty and Change* (Boston, MA: Shambhala Publications, 2013).

7. Mark Williams, John Teasdale, Zindel Segal, and Jon Kabat-Zinn, *The Mindful Way through Depression: Freeing Yourself from Chronic Unhappiness* (New York: The Guildford Press, 2007).

8. Kristen Neff, *Self-Compassion: The Proven Power of Being Kind to Yourself* (New York: Harper Collins, 2011).

9. Christopher K. Germer, *The Mindful Path to Self-Compassion: Freeing Yourself from Destructive Thoughts and Emotions* (New York: The Guilford Press, 2009).

CHAPTER 9

1. Andrea Chisholm MD, "Menopause Treatments," October 18, 2016, http://www.verywellhealth.menopause.about.com.treatment.

2. Christiane Northrup, MD, *The Wisdom of Menopause* (New York: Bantam Books, 2012).

3. Mia Lundin, *Female Brain Gone Insane* (Deerfield Beach, FL: Health Communications Inc., 2009).

4. Christiane Northrup, MD, "Do You Need Bioidentical Hormones?" September 11, 2017, https://www.drnorthrup.com/do-you-need-bioidentical-hormones.

5. Christiane Northrup, MD, "Herbs to Relieve Menopause Symptoms," September 11, 2017, https://www.drnorthrup.com/traditional-herbs-or-bioidentical-hormones-which-is-better.

6. James Francis Carmody, Sybil Crawford, Elena Salmoirago-Blotcher, Katherine Leung, Linda Churchill, and Nicholas Olendzki,

"Mindfulness Training for Coping with Hot Flashes," *Menopause* 18, no. 6 (2011): 611–20.

7. Northrup, *Wisdom of Menopause*.

8. Judith A. Houck, *Hot and Bothered: Women, Medicine, and Menopause in Modern America* (Cambridge, MA: Harvard University Press, 2006).

9. Heather E. Dillaway, "Menopause Is the 'Good Old': Women's Thoughts about Reproductive Aging," *Gender and Society* 19, no. 3 (June 2005): 398–417.

10. Julie A. Winterich, "Sex, Menopause, and Culture: Sexual Orientation and the Meaning of Menopause for Women's Sex Lives," *Gender and Society* 17, no. 4 (August 2003): 627–42.

11. Gail Sheehy, *The Silent Passage Menopause* (New York: Pocket Books, 2010).

12. Rebecca Skloot, *The Immortal Life of Henrietta Lacks* (New York: Crown Publishing Group, 2010).

13. Catherine Roberts, "8 Acupuncture Benefits for Menopausal Women," February 14, 2014, http://www.activebeat.com/Health/Women /8-acupuncture-benefits-for-menopausal-women.

14. Carmody et al., "Mindfulness Training."

15. Sharon Begley, *Train Your Mind, Change Your Brain* (New York: Ballantine Books, 2007).

16. Richard J. Davidson with Sharon Begley, *The Emotional Life of Your Brain* (New York: Plume, 2013).

17. Lundin, *Female Brain Gone Insane*.

18. Daniel J. Siegel, *Mindsight: The New Science of Personal Transformation* (New York: Bantam Books, 2010).

19. Mayo Clinic Staff, "Male Menopause: Myth or Reality?" https://www .mayoclinic.org/healthy-lifestyle/mens-health/in-depth/male-menopause.

APPENDIX B

1. This material comes from a conference entitled "Zen and the Art of Dealing with Difficult Emotions," taught by Reverend Steve Kanji Ruhl at the Rowe Camp and Conference Center in Rowe, Massachusetts, January 25–27, 2019.

2. Tara Brach, *True Refuge: Finding Peace and Freedom in Your Own Awakened Heart* (New York: Bantam Books, 2013).

3. Ibid.

4. Tsultrim Allione, *Feeding Your Demons: Ancient Wisdom for Resolving Inner Conflict* (New York: Little, Brown, and Company, 2008).

APPENDIX C

1. This material comes from a conference entitled "Befriending the Enemy: Liberating Yourself from Shadow Projections," taught by Polly Young-Eisendrath, Rowe Camp and Conference Center, Rowe, Massachusetts, February 15–18, 2019.

2. Polly Young-Eisendrath, *Love Between Equals: Relationship as a Spiritual Path* (Boulder, CO: Shambhala Publications, 2019).

3. Ibid., p. 88.

4. Ibid., p. 94.

5. Ibid., p. 108.

Bibliography

Anil, Bindhu S., Bhaskar Anitha, and Joseph Jose. "Prevalence of Menopausal Symptoms among Women (Menopausal < 5 years) in a Rural Area in Kottayam, Kerala, India." *Journal of Evolution of Medical and Dental Sciences* 3, no. 17 (April 28, 2014): 4648–60.

Baraz, James, and Shoshana Alexander. *Awakening Joy*. Berkeley, CA: Parallax Press, 2012.

Basaria, S., A. Wisniewski, K. Dupree, T. Bruno, M. Y. Song, F. Yao, A. Ojumu, M. John, and A. S. Dobs. "Effect of High-Dose Isoflavones on Cognition, Quality of Life, Androgens, and Lipoprotein in Post-Menopausal Women." *Journal of Endocrinological Investigation* 32, no. 2 (2009): 150–55.

Begley, Sharon. *Train Your Mind, Change Your Brain: How a New Science Reveals Our Extraordinary Potential to Transform Ourselves*. New York: Ballantine Books, 2007.

Bodenheimer, Thomas, and Kevin Grumbach. "Paying for Health Care." In *The Sociology of Health and Illness*, edited by Peter Conrad and Valerie Leiter, 9th ed., 326–36. New York: Worth Publishers, 2013.

Boston Women's Health Book Collective. *Our Bodies, Ourselves: Menopause*. New York: Simon and Schuster, 2006.

Boston Women's Health Book Collective and Judy Norsigian. *Our Bodies, Ourselves*. New York: Simon and Schuster, 2011.

Brach, Tara. *True Refuge: Finding Peace and Freedom in Your Own Awakened Heart*. New York: Bantam Books, 2013.

Breheny, M., and C. Stephens. "Healthy Living and Keeping Busy: A Discourse Analysis of Mid-Aged Women's Attributions for Menopausal Experience." *Journal of Language and Social Psychology* 22, no. 2 (2003): 169–89.

Brody, Jane E. "The Stubborn Markers of Menopause." *The New York Times* (February 11, 2014): Section D, 5.

Bromberger, Joyce T., Peter M. Meyer, Howard M. Kravitz, Barbara Sommer, Adriana Cordal, Lynda Powell, Patricia A. Ganz, and Kim Sutton-Tyrell. "Psychologic Distress and Natural Menopause: A Multiethnic Community Study." *American Journal of Public Health* 91, no. 9 (September 2001): 1435–42.

Carmody, James Francis, Sybil Crawford, Elena Salmoirago-Blotcher, Katherine Leung, Linda Churchill, and Nicholas Olendzki. "Mindfulness Training for Coping with Hot Flashes." *Menopause* 18, no. 6 (2011): 611–20.

Cayton, Karuna. *The Misleading Mind: How We Create Our Own Problems and How Buddhist Psychology Can Help Us Solve Them.* Novato, CA: New World Library, 2012.

Centers for Disease Control. "Leading Cause of Death in Females in the United States." 2015. https://www.cdc.gov/women/lcod/index.htm.

Centre for Menstrual Cycle and Ovulation Research. 2018. www.cmcor.ubc.ca/resources.

Chisholm, Andrea, MD. "Menopause Symptoms and Diagnosis." October 18, 2016. https://www.verywellhealth.Menopause.about.com.

Cho, Jeena. "The Science behind How Mindfulness Helps You to Break Negative Thought Patterns." *Forbes Magazine*. December 27, 2016. http://www.forbes.com/sites/jeenacho/2016/12/27/the-science-behind-how-mindfulness-helps-you-to-break-negative-thought-patterns/#3a0e0482f83a.

Chödrön, Pema. *Living Beautifully with Uncertainty and Change.* Boston, MA: Shambhala Publications, 2013.

Chödrön, Pema. *The Places That Scare You: A Guide to Fearlessness in Difficult Times.* Boulder, CO: Shambhala Publications, 2002.

Conrad, Peter, and Valerie Leiter. "From Lydia Pinkham to Queen Levitra: Direct-to-Consumer Advertising and Medicalization." In *The Sociology of Health and Illness*, edited by Peter Conrad and Valerie Leiter, 9th ed., 301–11. New York: Worth Publishers, 2013.

Cosmopolitan Staff. "Oh, What a Lovely Pill!" *Cosmopolitan* (July 1965): 33–37.

Creswell, J. David, and Emily K. Lindsay. "How Does Mindfulness Training Affect Health? A Mindfulness Stress Buffering Account." *Current Directions in Psychological Science* 23 (2014): 401–7.

Dammery, Sally. *First Blood: A Cultural Study of Menarche.* Clayton, Victoria, Australia: Monash University Publishing, 2016.

Davidson, R. J., J. Kabat-Zinn, J. Schumacher, M. Rosenkranz, D. Muller, and S. Santorelli. "Alterations in Brain and Immune Function Produced by Mindfulness Meditation." *Psychosomatic Medicine* 65, no. 4 (2003): 564–70.

Davidson, Richard J., with Sharon Begley. *The Emotional Life of Your Brain*. New York: Plume, 2013.

Delanoe, Daniel, Selma Jajri, Annie Bachelot, Dorra Mahfoudh Draoui, Danielle Hassoun, Elise Marsicano, and Virginie Ringa. "Class, Gender, and Culture in the Experience of Menopause: A Comparative Study in Tunisia and France." *Social Science and Medicine* 75 (2012): 401–9.

Diamond, L. M. *Sexual Fluidity: Understanding Women's Love and Desire*. Cambridge, MA: Harvard University Press, 2008.

Dillaway, Heather E. "Menopause Is the 'Good Old': Women's Thoughts about Reproductive Aging." *Gender and Society* 19, no. 3 (June 2005): 398–417.

Dillaway, Heather E. *Sex for Life: From Virginity to Viagra: How Sexuality Changes throughout Our Lives*. New York: NYU Press, 2012.

Dillaway, Heather E. "(Un)Changing Menopausal Bodies: How Women Think and Act in the Face of Reproductive Transition and Gendered Beauty Ideals." *Sex Roles* 53, no. 1/2 (July 2005): 1–17.

Dillaway, Heather E. "Why Can't You Control This? How Women's Interactions with Intimate Partners Define Menopause and Family." *Journal of Women and Aging* 20, no. 1 (2008): 47–64.

Dillaway, Heather E., and Mary Byrnes. "Talking 'Among Us': Racial and Ethnic Perspectives of the Menopausal Experience." Paper presented at the annual meetings of the American Sociological Association, Montreal, Canada, August 2006.

Elavsly, Steriani, and Edward McAuley. "Physical Activity, Symptoms, Esteem, and Life Satisfaction during Menopause." *Maturitas* 52, no. 3–4 (2005): 374–85.

Feng, Zhao. "Construction of Menopause: An Inquiry of Cultural Influences on Menopause and Associated Problems." Paper presented at the annual meetings of the American Sociological Association, Atlanta, Georgia, August 16, 2003.

Fielder, Katherine Vaughn, and Sharon E. Robinson Kurpius. "Marriage, Stress, and Menopause: Midlife Challenges and Joys." *Psicologia* 19, no. 1–2 (2005): 87–106.

Fletcher, Jenna. "Bioidentical Hormones: How Are They Used?" *Medical News Today.* September 19, 2017. http://medicalnewstoday.com /articles/319465.php.

Friedan, Betty. *The Fountain of Age.* New York: Simon and Schuster, 1993.

Garland, E. L., S. A. Gaylord, and B. L. Fredrickson. "Positive Reappraisal Mediates the Stress-Reductive Effects of Mindfulness: An Upward Spiral Process." *Mindfulness* 2 (2011): 59–67.

Gavrilov, L. A., and N. S. Gravrilova. "New Findings on Human Longevity Predictors." Paper presented at the Annual Meeting of the Gerontological Society of America, San Francisco, California, November 19, 2007.

Germer, Christopher K. *The Mindful Path to Self-Compassion.* New York: The Guilford Press, 2009.

Goldberg, Simon B., Raymond P. Tucker, Preston A. Greene, David J. Kearney, and Tracy L. Simpson. "Mindfulness-Based Interventions for Psychiatric Disorders: A Systematic Review and Meta-Analysis." *Clinical Psychology Review* 59 (February 2018): 52–60.

Gottfried, Sara, MD, and Christiane Northrup, MD (foreword). *The Hormone Cure: Reclaim Balance, Sleep, and Sex Drive: Lose Weight, Feel Focused, Vital and Energized Naturally with the Gottfried Protocol.* New York: Scribner, 2014.

Hahn, Thich Nhat. *The Heart of the Buddha's Teaching: Transforming Suffering into Peace, Joy, and Liberation.* New York: Harmony Books, 2015.

Hart, Vicki, Susan R. Sturgeon, Nicholas Reich, Lynnette Leidy Sievert, Sybil L. Crawford, and Ellen B. Gold. "Menopausal Vasomotor Symptoms and Incident Breast Cancer Risk in the Study of Women's Health across the Nation." *Cancer Causes and Control* 27, no. 11 (November 2016): 1333.

Hartmann, U., S. Philippsohn, K. Heiser, and C. Ruffer-Hess. "Low Sexual Desire in Midlife and Older Women: Personality Factors, Psychosocial Development, Present Sexuality." *Menopause* 11, no. 6 (2004): 726–40.

Harvard Health Letter. April 30, 2018. www.health.harvard.edu/mind-and -mood/exercise-is-an-all-natural-treatment-to-fight-depression.

Hendel, Amy. Reviewed by Peter J. Chen, MD, FACOG. "Ten Things You Should Know about Menopause." HealthCentral.com. November 2, 2012.

Herbalist Report. "Menopause Support Report 2017." 2017. www
.herbalistreport.com/menopause-herbal-solutions-bing/index2.html

Holzel, B. K., S. W. Lazar, T. Gard, Z. Schuman-Olivier, D. R. Vago, and
U. Ott. "How Does Mindfulness Meditation Work? Proposing
Mechanisms of Action from a Conceptual and Neural Perspec-
tive." *Perspectives on Psychological Science* 6 (2011): 537–59.

Houck, Judith A. *Hot and Bothered: Women, Medicine, and Menopause in
Modern America.* Cambridge, MA: Harvard University Press, 2006.

Kaufman, Sherwin A. "The Truth about Female Hormones." *Ladies Home
Journal* (January 1965): 22–23.

Kleinman, Arthur. *The Illness Narratives: Suffering, Healing, and the
Human Condition.* New York: Basic Books, 1998.

Kurpius, Sharon E. Robinson, Megan Foley Nicpon, and Susan E. Maresh.
"Mood, Marriage, and Menopause." *Journal of Counseling Psychology* 48, no. 1 (2001): 77–84.

Lazar, S., C. Kerr, R. Wasserman, J. Gray, D. Greve, M. Treadway, et al.
"Meditation Experience Is Associated with Increased Cortical
Thickness." *NeuroReport* 16, no. 17 (2005): 1893–97.

Lee, John R., and Virginia Hopkins. *What Your Doctor May Not Tell You
about Menopause: The Breakthrough Book on Natural Hormone
Balance.* New York: Warner Books, 2004.

Li, Alison. "Marketing Menopause: Science and the Public Relations of
Premarin." In *Women, Health and Nation: Canada and the United
States Since 1945*, edited by Georgina Feldberg, Molly Ladd-
Taylor, Alison Li, and Kathryn McPherson, 101–20. Montreal,
Quebec, Canada: McGill-Queen's University Press, 2003.

Lindau, Stacy Tessler, L. Philip Schumm, Edward O. Laumann, Wendy
Levinson, Colm Muircheartaigh, and Linda J. Waite. "A Study of
the Sexuality and Health among Older Adults in the United
States." *New England Journal of Medicine* 357 (2007): 762–74.

Lindsay, Emily K., and J. David Creswell. "Back to Basics: How Attention
Monitoring and Acceptance Stimulate Positive Growth." *Psychological Inquiry* 26 (2015): 343–48.

Lorber, Judith. *Gender and the Social Construction of Illness.* Thousand
Oaks, CA: Sage Publications, 1997.

Lundin, Mia. *Female Brain Gone Insane.* Deerfield Beach, FL: Health
Communications Inc., 2009.

Mayo Clinic. 2018. https://www.mayoclinic.org/diseases-conditions/meno
pause.

Mayo Clinic. July 24, 2018. https://www.mayoclinic.org/diseases-condi tions/endometriosis.

Mayo Clinic Staff. "Male Menopause: Myth or Reality?" 2017. https://www.mayoclinic.org/healthy-lifestyle/mens-health/in-depth/male -menopause.

Mindful Staff. "Jon Kabat-Zinn: Defining Mindfulness." January 11, 2017. www.mindful.org.

Moffitt, Phillip. *Emotional Chaos to Clarity: Move from the Chaos of the Reactive Mind to the Clarity of the Responsive Mind.* New York: Plume, 2013.

Moody, Harry R., and Jennifer R. Sasser. *Aging Concepts and Controversies.* Los Angeles, CA: Sage Publications, 2015.

Morrison, Lynn A., Lynnette L. Sievert, Daniel E. Brown, Nichole Rahberg, and Angela Reza. "Relationships between Menstrual and Menopausal Attitudes and Associated Demographic and Health Characteristics: The Hilo Women's Health Study." *Women and Health* 50 (2010): 397–413.

Neff, Kristen. *Self-Compassion: The Proven Power of Being Kind to Yourself.* New York: Harper Collins, 2011.

Newhart, Michelle R. "Menopause Matters: The Implications of Menopause Research for Studies of Midlife Health." *Health Sociology Review* 22, no. 4 (2013): 365–76.

Newsweek. "No More Menopause." *Newsweek* (January 13, 1964): 53.

Niemiec, Ryan M. "3 Definitions of Mindfulness That Might Surprise You." *Psychology Today.* November 1, 2017. https://www .psychologytoday.com.

Northrup, Christiane, MD. "Do You Need Bioidentical Hormones?" September 11, 2017. https://www.drnorthrup.com/do-you-need-bio identical-hormones.

Northrup, Christiane, MD. "Herbs to Relieve Menopause Symptoms." September 11, 2017. https://www.drnorthrup.com/traditional-herbs -or-bioidentical-hormones-which-is-better.

Northrup, Christiane, MD. *The Wisdom of Menopause,* 3rd ed. New York: Bantam Books, 2012.

Oakes, Kari. "Chronic Insomnia Affects One-Third in Perimenopause." *Clinical Psychiatry News* 44, no. 1 (January 2016): 27.

Office for National Statistics. "How Has Life Expectancy Changed over Time?" September 9, 2015. http://www.visual.ons.gov.uk/how-has -life-expectancy-changed-over-time.

Piver, Susan. *Start Here Now: An Open-Hearted Guide to the Path and Practice of Meditation*. Boston, MA: Shambhala, 2015.

Reuben, David. *Everything You Wanted to Know about Sex: But Were Afraid to Ask*. New York: David McKay Co., 1969.

Rimma, Teper, Zindel V. Segal, and Michael Inzlicht. "Inside the Mindful Mind: How Mindfulness Enhances Emotion Regulation through Improvements in Executive Control." *Current Directions in Psychological Science* 22 (2013): 449–54.

Ring, Melinda. *The Natural Menopause Solution: Expert Advice for Melting Stubborn Midlife Pounds, Reducing Hot Flashes, and Getting Relief from Menopause Symptoms*. New York: Rodale Books, 2012.

Roberts, Catherine. "8 Acupuncture Benefits for Menopausal Women." February 14, 2014. http://www.activebeat.com/Health/Women/8-acupuncture-benefits-for-menopausal-women.

Sheehy, Gail. *Passages: Predictable Crises of Adult Life*, 4th ed. New York: Ballantine Books, An Imprint of Random House, 2006.

Sheehy, Gail. *The Silent Passage: Menopause*, 6th ed. New York: Pocket Books, An Imprint of Simon and Schuster Inc., 1991, 2010.

Shifren, J. L., B. U. Monz, P. A. Russo, A. Segreti, and C. B. Johannes. "Sexual Problems and Distress in United States Women: Prevalence and Correlates." *Obstetrics and Gynecology* 112 (2008): 970–78.

Siegel, Daniel J. *Aware: The Science and Practice of Presence*. New York: TarcherPerigee, 2018.

Siegel, Daniel J. *Mindsight: The New Science of Personal Transformation*. New York: Bantam Books, 2010.

Sievert, Lynette Leidy. *Menopause: A Biocultural Perspective*. Rutgers, NJ: Rutgers University Press, 2006.

Skloot, Rebecca. *The Immortal Life of Henrietta Lacks*. New York: Crown Publishing Group, 2010.

Song, Sora. "Examining 'Male Menopause': Myth or Malady?" Time.com. June 16, 2010. http://healthland.time.com/2010/06/16/examining-the-myth-of-male-menopause/print.

Sontag, Susan. *Illness as Metaphor and AIDS and Its Metaphors*. New York: Picador, 2001.

Spettel, Sarah, and Mark Donald White. "The Portrayal of J. Marion Sims' Controversial Surgical Legacy." *The Journal of Urology* 185 (June 2011): 2424–27.

Strauss, Judy R. "The Baby Boomers Meet Menopause: Fertility, Attractiveness, and Affective Response to the Menopausal Transition." *Sex Roles* 68 (2013): 77–90.

Strauss, Judy R. "Contextual Influences on Women's Health Concerns and Attitudes towards Menopause." *Health and Social Work* 36, no. 2 (May 2011): 121–27.

Tang, Yi-Yuan, Britta K. Holzel, and Michael I. Posner. "The Neuroscience of Mindfulness Meditation." *Nature Reviews Neuroscience* 16 (March 18, 2015): 213–25.

Utz, Rebecca. "Like Mother, (Not) Like Daughter: The Social Construction of Menopause and Aging." *Journal of Aging Studies* 25 (2011): 143–54.

Vogue Staff. "How to Live Young at Any Age." *Vogue* (August 1965): 61–64.

Waehner, Paige. "Ease into Menopause with Exercise." 2016. http://www.verywell.com/ease-into-menopause-with-exercise-1231560.

Wall, L. L. "The Medical Ethics of Dr. J. Marion Sims: A Fresh Look at the Historical Record." *Journal of Medical Ethics* 32, no. 6 (June 2006): 346–50.

Walsh, Ann. *E.R.T.: The Pills to Keep Women Young.* New York: Bantam, 1965.

Walter, Carolyn Ambler. "The Psychosocial Meaning of Menopause: Women's Experiences." *Journal of Women and Aging* 12, no. 3/4 (2000): 117–31.

Whitely, Jennifer, Marco daCosta DiBonaventura, Jan-Samuel Wagner, Jose Alvir, and Sonali Shah. "The Impact of Menopausal Symptoms on Quality of Life, Productivity, and Economic Outcomes." *Journal of Women's Health* 22, no. 11 (2013): 983–90.

Williams, Mark, John Teasdale, Zindel Segal, and Jon Kabat-Zinn. *The Mindful Way through Depression.* New York: The Guilford Press, 2007.

Wilson, D. "Drug for Sexual Disorder Opposed by Panel." *The New York Times* (June 19, 2010): B3. Available online at www.nytimes.com/2010/06/19/business/19sexpill.html.

Wilson, Robert A., and Thelma A. Wilson. "The Fate of the Nontreated Postmenopausal Woman: A Plea for the Maintenance of Adequate Estrogen from Puberty to the Grave." *Journal of the American Geriatrics Society* 11 (1963): 347–62.

Wilson, Robert A., and Thelma A. Wilson. *Feminine Forever.* New York: M. Evans and Company, 1966.

Wingert, Pat, and Barbara Kantrowitz. *The Menopause Book*, 2nd ed. New York: Workman Publishing, 2009.

Winterich, Julie A. "From Biology to Culture: The Roles of Gender, Race, and Sexuality for Women's Menopausal Experiences." Paper presented at the annual meetings of the American Sociological Society, Atlanta, Georgia, August 16, 2003.

Winterich, Julie A. "Sex, Menopause, and Culture: Sexual Orientation and the Meaning of Menopause for Women's Sex Lives." *Gender and Society* 17, no. 4 (August, 2003): 627–42.

Winterich, Julie A., and Debra Umberson. "How Women Experience Menopause: The Importance of Social Context." *Journal of Women and Aging* 11, no. 4 (1999): 57–73.

Women's Health Initiative. www.whi.org/about.

Writing Group for the Women's Health Initiative Investigation. "Risk and Benefits of Estrogen and Progestin in Healthy Postmenopausal Women." *Journal of the American Medical Association* 268 (2002): 321–33.

Zhang, Sarah. "The Surgeon Who Experimented on Slaves." *The Atlantic.* April 18, 2018.

Zhang, Shumin M., JoAnn E. Manson, Kathryn M. Rexrode, Nancy R. Cook, Julie E. Burning, and I-Min Lee. "Use of Oral Conjugated Estrogen Alone and Risk of Breast Cancer." *American Journal of Epidemiology* 165, no. 5 (March 1, 2007): 524–29.

Index

About the Author

Deborah M. Merrill, PhD, is professor of sociology and past associate dean, chair of the faculty, and chair of the steering committee at Clark University, Massachusetts, where she began teaching in 1992 as an assistant professor. She teaches courses on the sociology of medicine, families, aging, and methodology. She has authored four books as well as encyclopedia entries and articles published in the *Journal of Aging and Health*, *Research on Aging, Ethnic Groups, Social Forces, Journal of Social and Personal Relationships, Journal of Marriage and Family, Disabilities Studies Quarterly*, and *Contemporary Sociology*. Merrill has served as a reviewer for the *Journal of Marriage and Family, Journal of Family Issues, Journal of Family Theory and Review*, and the *Journal of Aging and Health*. Before launching her career, she held a postdoctoral fellowship at the Brown University Center for Gerontology and Health Care Research. Her previous book with Praeger/ABC-CLIO is *Mothers-in-Law and Daughters-in-Law: Understanding the Relationship and What Makes Them Friends or Foe.*